Applications of Ultrasound in Anesthesia
A Handbook

AF067351

Applications of Ultrasound in Anesthesia
A Handbook

Kavita S Lalchandani
MD DA (Anesthesiology) Fellow in Emergency Medicine

Associate Professor
Department of Anesthesiology
SSG Hospital and Medical College
Vadodara, Gujarat, India

Foreword
MR Upadhyay

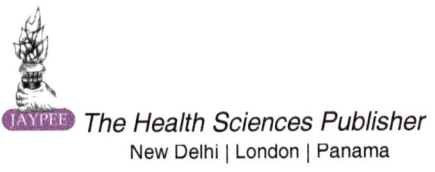

The Health Sciences Publisher
New Delhi | London | Panama

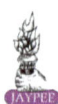

Jaypee Brothers Medical Publishers (P) Ltd

Headquarters

Jaypee Brothers Medical Publishers (P) Ltd
4838/24, Ansari Road, Daryaganj
New Delhi 110 002, India
Phone: +91-11-43574357
Fax: +91-11-43574314
Email: jaypee@jaypeebrothers.com

Overseas Offices

J.P. Medical Ltd
83 Victoria Street, London
SW1H 0HW (UK)
Phone: +44 20 3170 8910
Fax: +44 (0)20 3008 6180
Email: info@jpmedpub.com

Jaypee Brothers Medical Publishers (P) Ltd
17/1-B Babar Road, Block-B, Shaymali
Mohammadpur, Dhaka-1207
Bangladesh
Mobile: +08801912003485
Email: jaypeedhaka@gmail.com

Jaypee-Highlights Medical Publishers Inc
City of Knowledge, Bld. 235, 2nd Floor, Clayton
Panama City, Panama
Phone: +1 507-301-0496
Fax: +1 507-301-0499
Email: cservice@jphmedical.com

Jaypee Brothers Medical Publishers (P) Ltd
Bhotahity, Kathmandu
Nepal
Phone: +977-9741283608
Email: kathmandu@jaypeebrothers.com

Website: www.jaypeebrothers.com
Website: www.jaypeedigital.com

© 2018, Jaypee Brothers Medical Publishers

The views and opinions expressed in this book are solely those of the original contributor(s)/author(s) and do not necessarily represent those of editor(s) of the book.

All rights reserved. No part of this publication may be reproduced, stored or transmitted in any form or by any means, electronic, mechanical, photocopying, recording or otherwise, without the prior permission in writing of the publishers.

All brand names and product names used in this book are trade names, service marks, trademarks or registered trademarks of their respective owners. The publisher is not associated with any product or vendor mentioned in this book.

Medical knowledge and practice change constantly. This book is designed to provide accurate, authoritative information about the subject matter in question. However, readers are advised to check the most current information available on procedures included and check information from the manufacturer of each product to be administered, to verify the recommended dose, formula, method and duration of administration, adverse effects and contraindications. It is the responsibility of the practitioner to take all appropriate safety precautions. Neither the publisher nor the author(s)/editor(s) assume any liability for any injury and/or damage to persons or property arising from or related to use of material in this book.

This book is sold on the understanding that the publisher is not engaged in providing professional medical services. If such advice or services are required, the services of a competent medical professional should be sought.

Every effort has been made where necessary to contact holders of copyright to obtain permission to reproduce copyright material. If any have been inadvertently overlooked, the publisher will be pleased to make the necessary arrangements at the first opportunity. The **CD/DVD-ROM** (if any) provided in the sealed envelope with this book is complimentary and free of cost. **Not meant for sale**.

Inquiries for bulk sales may be solicited at: jaypee@jaypeebrothers.com

Applications of Ultrasound in Anesthesia: A Handbook

First Edition: **2018**

ISBN 978-93-5270-270-1

Dedicated to

His Holiness Sant Hirdaram Sahib ji

FOREWORD

Ultrasound technology is a rapidly emerging science with wide applications in the field of medicine. It is a safe, reliable, relatively inexpensive and portable imaging modality. It plays an important role in identifying the correct anatomy of underlying 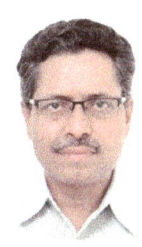 structures and has therefore served as a very good diagnostic tool in medical science.

Practice of anesthesia also requires the correct identification of anatomical landmarks for proper placement of drugs in regional anesthesia blocks given for anesthesia or analgesia purpose. In emergencies as well as in cases with difficult anatomy to locate the required landmarks, ultrasound serves as a rescue device. Current and future applications of ultrasound in the field of anesthesia include regional anesthesia, epidural space identification in cases of difficult anatomy, delineating nerve plexuses for chronic pain procedures, vascular access, airway assessment, lung ultrasound, ultrasound neuro-monitoring, gastric ultrasound, focused transthoracic echo (TTE), transesophageal echo (TEE) and Doppler. Airway assessment applications do include identification of cricothyroid membrane for cricothyrotomy in emergency as well as assessing the tracheal diameter for selecting the proper sized endotracheal tube particularly in small kids. Practice of ultrasound is gradually becoming routine in daily practice of anesthesia and pain management in many of the centers of India and is going to become common application everywhere. It is therefore a perfect time when young anesthesia postgraduate residents be made familiar with practice of ultrasound.

Applications of Ultrasound in Anesthesia: A Handbook has been written by Dr Kavita S Lalchandani with the purpose to explain the basics of ultrasound and its applications to young budding anesthesiologists in a very simple understandable language with diagrams and ultrasound photographs wherever required.

The initial chapters in this book deal with the knowledge of ultrasound which includes parts of ultrasound, terminologies and how to do scanning, while in other chapters the author has discussed ultrasound-guided procedures like central venous access and various regional blocks.

I am sure that the book will be appreciated by the anesthesia fraternity—both consultants and young students of anesthesiology and I wish it to become a regular handbook for them while carrying out a procedure in operation theater or in intensive care under ultrasound guidance.

MR Upadhyay
MD (Anesthesiology)
Senior Professor and Head
Department of Anaesthesiology
SSG Hospital and Government Medical College
Vadodara, Gujarat

Ex-President
Indian Society of Anesthesiologists
Gujarat State Branch

Ex-Chief-Editor
Gujarat Journal of Anesthesiology

Ex-Editor, Indian Journal of
Anesthesia and Analgesia

PREFACE

Future is all about advancement and ultrasound is one such advancement in medical practice. It is rapidly emerging science with wide applications in the field of medicine. It is a safe, reliable, relatively inexpensive and portable imaging modality. It plays an important role in identifying the correct anatomy of underlying structures and has therefore served as a very good diagnostic tool in medical science.

The book describes the basics of ultrasound, different terminologies used in ultrasound and simplified way of performing anesthetic procedures under ultrasound guidance.

Kavita S Lalchandani

ACKNOWLEDGMENTS

It is most appropriate that I begin by expressing my gratitude to the Almighty for having blessed me to write this book.

Any accomplishment requires the whole-hearted efforts (cooperation) of many people and this work is not different. This has been the result of teamwork put together by certain people without their support, encouragement and motivation this would not have seen the light of the day.

It gives me immense pleasure to express my deep gratitude, respect and sincere thanks to Dr MR Upadhyay, Senior Professor and Head, Department of Anesthesiology, SSG Hospital and Government Medical College, Vadodara, Gujarat for his advice and guidance and sharing his extraordinary experiences and unflinching encouragement throughout the work. His insight, high calibre and personal qualities have been profoundly inspirational to me.

I would like to thank Dr Neha Shah, Assistant Professor in Anesthesiology for her support in writing chapter 8: Transversus Abdominis Plane Block.

Above all, my sincere most appreciation goes to my husband Dr Shyam Lalchandani and my children for their unfailing motivation in all my academic endeavors and for their understanding, patience and encouragement during the long tedious hours of hard work amidst piles of papers and the glow of the computer screen.

My sincere thanks to Mr Sharad Patel whose dynamism to publish this book by M/s Jaypee Brothers Medical Publishers (P) Ltd, New Delhi, India, is a constant driving force for me to come out with this new book.

CONTENTS

Chapter 1. Basics of Ultrasound — 1
- Parts of the Ultrasound Machine 3
- Different Types of Ultrasound 7
- Selecting an Ultrasound Transducer Probe Based on Frequency, Array and Footprint 9
- Learning to Scan 11
- Artifacts 12
- Ultrasound Terminology 14

Chapter 2. Ultrasound-guided Central Venous Access — 16
- Basic Principles 18
- Indications and Contraindications 18
- Equipment Specifications 20
- General Protocol for Central Line Placement 21
- General Consideration for Ultrasound-guided Vascular Access 25
- Ultrasound-guided Vascular Access Line Placement 34
- Technique for Internal Jugular Vein Cannulation 36
- Technique for Subclavian Vein 44
- Technique for Femoral Vein Cannulation 48
- Alternative Central Venous Cannulation Sites 49
- Documentation 51

Chapter 3. Complications and their Management — 57
- Complications of Central Venous Access 57
- Infectious Complications of Central Venous Catheterization and their Prevention 58
- Mechanical Complications 60
- Management of Arterial Trauma or Injury due to Central Venous Catheterization 62
- Thrombotic Complications 63

Chapter 4. Ultrasound-guided Peripheral Venous Access — 66
- Peripheral Venous Access 66
- Technique for Ultrasound-guided Peripheral Venous Access 68

Chapter 5. Introduction of Ultrasound-guided Regional Block — 75
- History 75
- Local Anesthetic Agents 76
- Regional Anesthesia 78
- Ultrasound-guided Regional Blocks 83

Chapter 6. Upper Extremity Nerve Blocks — 86
- Brachial Plexus Block 87
- Ultrasound-guided Forearm Block 103

Chapter 7. Lower Extremity Nerve Blocks — 110
- Ultrasound-guided Femoral Nerve Block 110
- Ultrasound-guided Popliteal Sciatic Nerve Block 113

Chapter 8. Transversus Abdominis Plane Block — 119
- Anatomy 119
- Indications 121
- The Landmark Technique for TAP Block 122
- Ultrasound-guided TAP Block 122
- Ultrasound Anatomy 122
- Technique of TAP Block 125
- Complications 129

Index 131

Chapter 1

Basics of Ultrasound

INTRODUCTION

What is Ultrasound?

Ultrasound (US) is basically a medical imaging technique that uses high frequency sound waves. Historically, medical ultrasound was born out of SONAR (Sound Navigation and Ranging) technology after World War II. As SONAR technology improved the ultrasound came into field as diagnostic imaging, using high-frequency sound waves and the pulse-echo principle to display normal and abnormal anatomy. Ultrasound has been used to image the human body for over half a century. Dr Karl Theo Dussik, an Austrian neurologist, was the first to apply ultrasound as a medical diagnostic tool to image the brain.

Nowadays, the role of ultrasound for anesthesiologist is mainly for vascular access and different regional blocks. The main goal of introduction of ultrasound techniques into anesthesia practice is to improve patient safety and interventional anesthesia efficacy.

In this chapter we are going to discuss about basic principles of ultrasound, US machine, basic terminology and sonographic view of different tissues.

The main principles of ultrasound are as follows:
- The machine first transmits high frequency pulse waves into body using probe and then these waves are reflected back to the probe
- From the probe waves are relayed to the machine
- The machine calculates the distance from the probe to the tissue or organ (boundaries) using the speed of sound in tissue (5,005 ft/s or 1,540 m/s) and the time of the each echo's return (usually on the order of millionths of a second)
- The machine displays the distances and intensities of the echoes on the screen, forming a two dimensional image.

Advantages of Ultrasound

- There are no radiation hazards with ultrasound machine. It is portable and cost-effective compared to other imaging modalities
- We can perform the procedure under ultrasound guidance at the same time while visualizing the targeted structure
- Using ultrasound we can visualize the targeted structure, the distribution of the injected medication, and the capacity to control its distribution by readjusting the needle position, if needed
- US guidance improves the success rate of the procedures, their safety and speed.
- In addition to bony tissue Ultrasound can also visualize soft tissue.

Disadvantages of Ultrasound

- While performing procedures under ultrasound guidance it is necessary to have a thorough knowledge of gross or microanatomy

- For the best use of US in acute pain medicine and regional anesthesia, one should memorize image of a targeted structure
- Thus, it requires lot of experience before doing procedure independently.

PARTS OF THE ULTRASOUND MACHINE (FIG. 1)

A basic ultrasound machine has the following parts:
- *Transducer probe:* Probe that sends and receives the sound waves.
- *Central processing unit (CPU):* Like other computers it is also considered as brain of the Ultrasound machine, which does all of the calculations.
- *Transducer pulse controls:* Changes the amplitude, frequency and duration of the pulses emitted from the transducer probe.
- *Display:* It is a screen on which all the processed images are displayed.

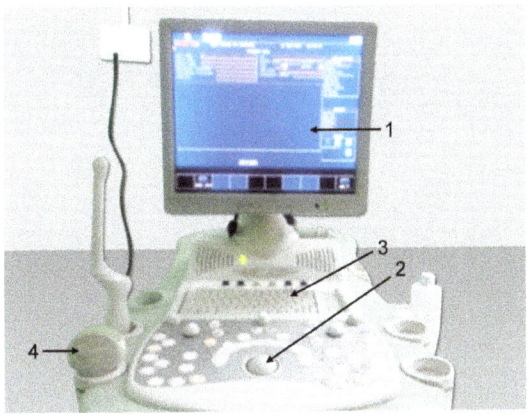

Fig. 1: Showing ultrasound machine and parts of machine: 1. Display screen, 2. Cursor, 3. Keyboard, 4. Transducer (curvilinear)

- *Keyboard/cursor:* Keyboard is used to enter the patient's data and to take necessary measurements of images from the display.
- *Disc storage device (hard, floppy, CD):* Is a storage unit of contained data.
- *Printer:* Printer is used to take the hard copies of acquired images.

Transducer Probe

The main part of the machine is transducer probe. The Transducer probes come in different shapes, depending on what structures are to be visualized (Fig. 2). Two main transducer probes are curvilinear and rectangular.

The rectangular probe also known as linear probe has high frequency which is useful to visualize superficial structures close to the skin surface (Fig. 3). While curvilinear probe has low frequency and used to visualize deeper structures like liver and gallbladder.

The transducer has orientation marker which correlates with a specific indicator on display.

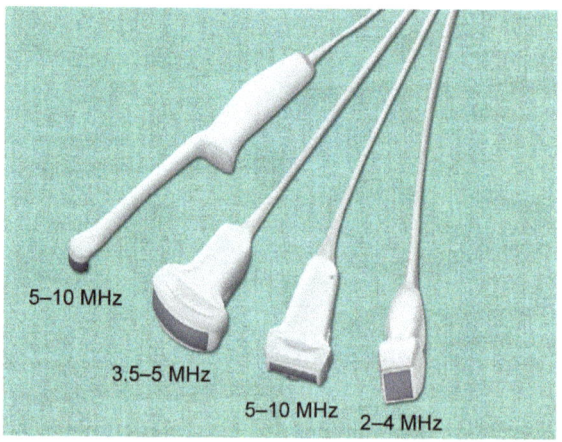

Fig. 2: Different types of transducers

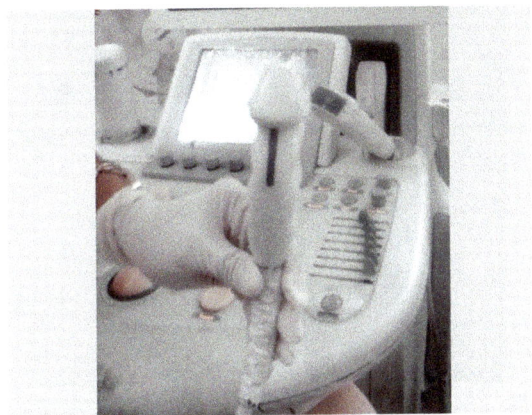

Fig. 3: Orientation marker of linear transducer probe

Usually orientation marker on display is kept on left side of the person performing the procedure.

Central Processing Unit

As in computer central processing unit (CPU) is the brain of the ultrasound machine. It contains the microprocessor, amplifier, transducer and memory unit with power supply. The CPU does all of the calculations involved in processing the data, and then forms the image on the monitor. The CPU also stores the processed data and/or image on disc.

Transducer Pulse Controls

It is useful to set and change the frequency and duration of the ultrasound pulses.

Ultrasound Knobology (Fig. 4)

Ultrasound machine has following buttons.
- *On-Off*: It is used when we first start the machine.

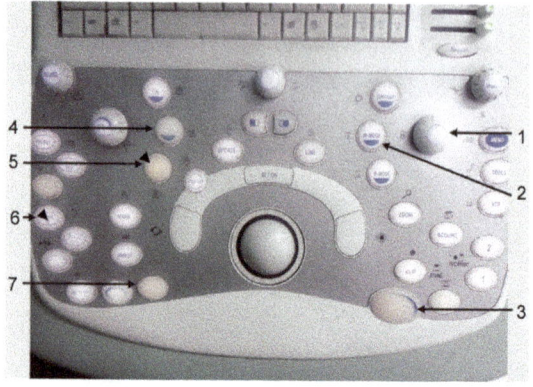

Fig. 4: Knobology of ultrasound machine: 1. Gain knob, 2. M-mode, 3. Freeze button, 4. Pulse wave button, 5. Color flow button, 6. Probe preset, 7. Measurement button

- *Probe preset:* This button is used to select the probe.
- *Depth:* This button is used to adjust the depth of the image. When we start scanning we should start with higher depth setting to get big picture and then decrease gradually till we get the targeted structure. Usually depth should be set at around 1 cm deeper than targeted structure.
- *Focus:* This button is used to set the focus of the image.
- *Gain:* Controls overall brightness of the image. When we change the gain it will change the amount of white, black, and gray of image on the monitor. This helps operator to distinguish structures on the screen.
- *Freeze:* Once you get the image properly you can view it by freezing the image.

Time Gain Compensation (TGC)

- *Frequency:* We can change the frequency of transducer probe according to depth of targeted structure.
- *Measurements:* This is one of the important tools to measure the distance of various images.

- *Color Doppler:* It is helpful to confirm the vessels.
- *Power Doppler:* It is used to differentiate artery from vein.
- *M-mode:* This is particularly useful when we want to see the images in motion, e.g. when we are giving supraclavicular brachial plexus block M-mode helps to prevent accidental pleura puncture by visualizing breathing movement.
- *Print/Save:* The machine can save and print the acquired images.

Display

The display screen shows the image of targeted structure and processed data from the CPU. It can be black and white or color.

Keyboard/Cursor

As in computer Ultrasound machine also has a keyboard and a cursor, such as a trackball, built in which help to add the patient data and to take measurements from the data.

Disc Storage

If we want to store the patient data or images we can store it in disc storage so that it can be useful for future references.

Printers

Printers are used to take out hard copy of the image from display.

DIFFERENT TYPES OF ULTRASOUND

1. *Two-dimensional imaging:* The above features which we have discussed will present two-dimensional images.

2. *3D ultrasound imaging:* Machines capable of three dimensional imaging have been developed recently.
3. *Doppler ultrasound:* Doppler ultrasound is useful to measure the rate of blood flow.

Imaging Modalities

- *B-mode (Brightness mode):* Displays a two-dimensional image.
- *M-mode (Motion mode):* It is a motion mode that means we can visualize moving objects in ultrasound. Particularly useful to anesthesiologist during vascular access and block to confirm the position of pleura and lung thereby preventing complications like pneumothorax as well as to evaluate for pneumothorax.
- Doppler is primarily used to detect blood flow and to assess direction and velocity.
- Color Doppler is useful to identify the presence and direction of flow as shown in Figure 5
- Pulse wave Doppler is used to confirm the artery as shown in Figure 6.

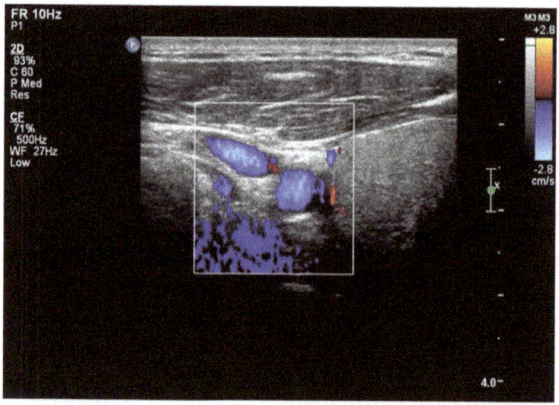

Fig. 5: Color Doppler used to confirm the anechoic vessel

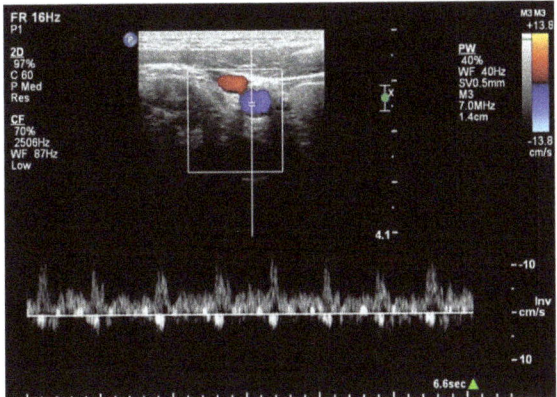

Fig. 6: Pulse wave Doppler showing artery is pulsatile (Blue). In US it is not necessary that artery is seen red and vein blue, it depends on the flow of the vessel. Blue away from the transducer and red towards the transducer

Appearance of Various Body Tissues on Ultrasound

Various body tissues appear differently on ultrasound. Some tissues absorb sound waves while some reflects them.

So, *Fluid* is always seen *Black* and *Tissue→Gray*. Thus, the denser the tissue, brighter white it appears in ultrasound. The bone appears brightest white (Fig. 7).

SELECTING AN ULTRASOUND TRANSDUCER PROBE BASED ON FREQUENCY, ARRAY AND FOOTPRINT

Frequency

- Frequency is a key property of each transducer. They are broadly categorized as high, mid, and low-frequency transducers

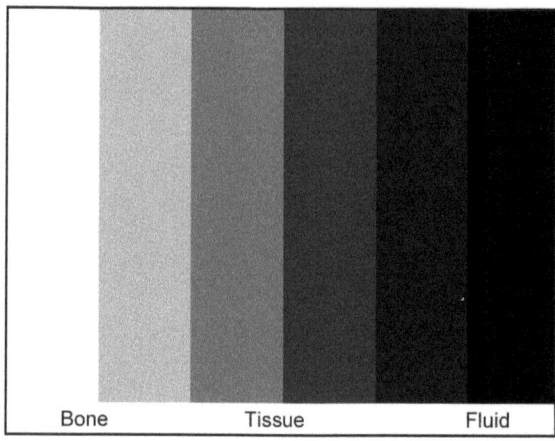

Fig. 7: Appearance of various body tissues on ultrasound

- *High frequency transducers:* High frequency transducers usually operate above 10 MHz and are mainly used to visualize structures less than 3 cm from the surface of the skin. These transducers are commonly used for examination of superficial structures such as peripheral nerves, or superficial vessels
- *'Mid-range' transducers (5-10 MHz):* Mid frequency transducers are used to visualize structures at approximately 3-6 cm below the skin surface like infraclavicular brachial plexus, sciatic nerve, or deeper vascular structures
- *'Low frequency' transducers (below 5 MHz):* Low frequency transducers are used to visualize deeper structures like liver, spleen and other body organs. These are also useful for performing procedures in obese patients.

Array Configuration

- Array means arrangement of elements on the face of the transducer. There are mainly two array configurations, (1) linear and (2) curved
- Basically linear arrays have flat surface which can provide anatomical visualization of the same width at the skin surface thereby providing uniform visualization of the image. The linear array transducers are useful mainly to anesthesiologist for visualizing superficial structures like vessels and nerve
- The transducers that have curved surface provide wide area of anatomical field. Curved array transducers are used for visualizing the deeper structures. These are particularly useful when superficial structures are obscuring the view of deeper structure of interest.

LEARNING TO SCAN

The most important part in Ultrasound is how to start the scanning. First we choose the transducer according to structure of interest. The four things are important in scanning.

1. *Pressure:* Pressure must be applied evenly to get the correct direction of the scan; however, sometimes more pressure may be required in order to direct the US beam in the desired manner (angling the probe). When viewing vessel pressure is also applied to compress a vein or to push an anatomical structure out of the way of an intended needle pass. But excessive pressure can cause discomfort to the patient.
2. *Sliding:* We use sliding to find the structure of interest and position it optimally on the screen. This is particularly required when we are using out of plan

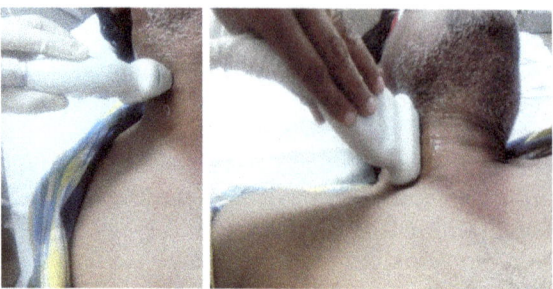

Fig. 8: Showing rotation of transducer from out of plane to in plane

approach where we bring the image in center of the screen.
3. *Rotation:* Usually we rotate the transducer to change the plane of interrogation, e.g. when we want to change from out of plane to in plane as shown in Figure 8.
4. *Tilt:* Tilting the probe is required when we do not get the desired image.

ARTIFACTS

Sometimes apart from desired image other different image may be seen which may not directly correlate with actual tissue, but may be helpful in diagnostic and procedural ultrasound. Usually three types of artifacts are seen: reverberation, refraction, and acoustic shadowing.
1. *Reverberation (Fig. 9):* Reverberation artifact appears as multiple reflection or echoes which gradually weakens. It is an artifactual image caused by delay of an echo that has been reflected back and forward again before returning to the transducer. They are usually seen posterior to the needle during procedure (e.g. While cannulating central line through out of plane approach tip of the needle can be seen as reverberation artifact)

Basics of Ultrasound

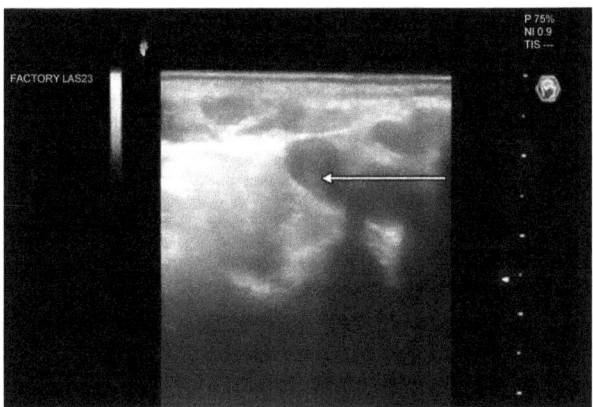

Fig. 9: Showing ring down reverberation artifact

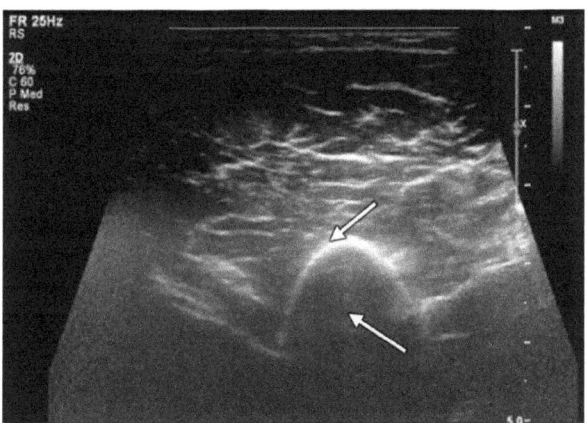

Fig. 10: Showing acoustic shadow bone appears as hyperechoic line below that acoustic shadow is seen

2. *Refraction artifact:* It is usually seen at the curve of a rounded object.
3. *Acoustic shadow (Fig. 10):* Mostly seen with highly attenuating structures like bone which cast an acoustic shadow immediately deep to the structure.

ULTRASOUND TERMINOLOGY (FIG. 11)

- *Echogenicity:* Echogenicity means appearance of the structure in the context of surrounding tissue Various body tissues conduct sound differently. Some tissues absorb sound waves while others reflect them. Thus, *Fluid* is always *Black* and *Tissue* is *Gray*. The denser the tissue, is the brighter white it will appear in ultrasound, the bone appears brightest white.
- *Three terminologies are used:*
  1. **Hyperechoic:** Structure appears white on the screen.
  2. **Hypoechoic:** Structure appears gray on the screen.
  3. **Anechoic:** Structure appears black on the screen.

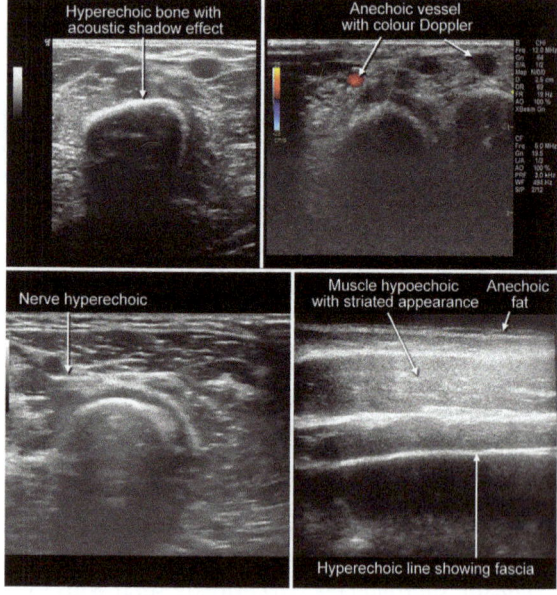

Fig. 11: Showing different structures according to ultrasound terminologies

Identifying structures according to above terminologies:

Bone	Bright rim with acoustic shadow
Cartilage	Hypoechoic
Vessel	*Black or anechoic:* Veins are usually easily collapsible upon external pressure by the transducer, while arteries are pulsatile and do not collapse with moderate pressure. Can be confirmed by color Doppler mode
Nerve	*Variable:* Proximal nerves—hypoanechoic (approximately similar to blood vessels but neither collapsible nor pulsatile); distal nerves: hyperechoic, with a stippled (honeycomb) structure
Lymph nodes	Anechoic or hypoechoic
Fascia	Hyperechoic lines
Fat	Anechoic
Muscles	Hypoechoic with striated structure
Lungs	Should be seen in M-mode hyperechoic pleura can be seen sliding in rhythm with each breath

BIBLIOGRAPHY

1. Chan V, Pearlas A. Basics of ultrasound imaging: 2011. pp.13-19.
2. Ihnatsenka B, Boezaart AP. Ultrasound: Basic understanding and learning the language. Int J Shoulder Surg. 2010;4(3):55-62.
3. Tirado A, Nagdev A, Henningsen C, Breckon P, Chiles K. Ultrasound guided procedures in the emergency department. Needle Guidance and Localization. 2013;31(1):87-115.
4. Vaughan B, Whitcomb MB, Maher O. How to Improve Accuracy of Ultrasound-Guided Procedures: American Association of Equine Practitioners Proceedings. 2009;55:438-48.

Chapter 2

Ultrasound-guided Central Venous Access

INTRODUCTION

Central venous pressure (CVP) is the pressure of blood in the thoracic vena cava, near the right atrium of the heart. CVP reflects the amount of blood returning to the heart and the ability of the heart to pump the blood into the arterial system.

Nowadays we are accessing veins and arteries to infuse fluids, medicines and blood products; for laboratory testing and invasive hemodynamic monitoring. These are the routine practice but, when the critically ill patient require more invasive access, monitoring, or aggressive resuscitation, central venous access is required instead of or in addition to peripheral venous access. Thus, central venous catheter allows one a stable, long-term access to large veins, and facilitates hemodynamic monitoring of the critically ill patient as well as route for the administration of multiple, sometimes vasoactive medications that cannot be given via peripheral veins.

Central venous access is defined as placement of a catheter such that the catheter is inserted into a venous great vessel. The main great vessels are the superior vena cava, inferior vena cava and brachiocephalic veins. Routinely we cannulate internal jugular veins, subclavian veins and femoral veins.

Now the question arises why procedure should be done under ultrasound guidance? As we all know very well that complications of central venous cannulation like arterial puncture, hematoma, air embolism and other mechanical complications are common with blind technique and such complications definitely can be reduced by performing procedure under ultrasound guidance. Again future is all about advancement and Ultrasound is one of such advancement. The role of ultrasound has expanded to such an extent in day to day practice that time will come when people will use it as audio visual stethoscope. So considering all these aspects this chapter includes

- Advantages and disadvantages of ultrasound
- Basic principles of central venous cannulation
- Indications and contraindications of central venous cannulation
- Specific indications for ultrasound guidance of central venous cannulation
- Equipment specification
- General protocol for central line placement
- General consideration for US guided vascular access
- US guided vascular access line placement
- Documentation.

Advantages of Ultrasound

- Using external landmarks for vascular access, there are high chances of complications like arterial puncture, pneumothorax, hematoma
- Bedside ultrasonography can be used to improve the ease, safety, and rapidity of access to both the arterial and venous systems
- Appropriately used ultrasound guidance for vascular access has been shown to reduce iatrogenic injury, improve effectiveness, reduce complications in diverse applications, reduce time and number of

attempts for successful cannulation. Additionally, it may improve patient comfort and satisfaction. It is like driving a car on 6 lane track.

Disadvantages

- It is a user dependent technology, before using it we should know the basics of the physics and instrumentation of ultrasound
- It requires hand-eye coordination for image acquisition and interpretation and lot of practice.

BASIC PRINCIPLES

- Put the central line only when it is really indicated
- Know the anatomy
- Be familiar with all equipment
- Obtain optimal patient positioning and consent
- Use sterile technique
- Always have a hand on your wire
- Ask for help
- Always aspirate as you advance the needle
- Always withdraw the needle to the level of the skin before redirecting the angle
- Obtain chest X-ray post line placement and review it.

INDICATIONS AND CONTRAINDICATIONS

Indications

- For patients who require hemodynamic monitoring, such as central venous pressure or a pulmonary artery catheter
- For procedures such as hemodialysis or transvenous pacing or for the administration of medications such as vasopressors, sclerosing medications, and cytotoxic and chemotherapeutic agents, TPN

- In the emergency setting, central venous access may be obtained during active resuscitation of critically ill patients
- In some cases, central venous access is used for patients in whom peripheral venous access cannot be gained.

Special Situations where Ultrasound is Useful

Ultrasound-guided CV access achieves its highest benefits in patients having:
- Morbid obesity
- Severe edema
- Uncorrected coagulopathy
- Multiple previous blind catheterizations
- History of prior failed CVC insertion
- Distorted anatomy
- Shock
- Burns
- Cardiac arrest.

Contraindications

When an experienced person is performing the procedure there are no absolute contraindications for CVP insertion, but contraindications for central venous access are relative and depend on the patient's status and the urgency of the procedure. General contraindications include:
- Bleeding disorders
- Anticoagulation or thrombolytic therapy
- Combative patients
- Distorted local anatomy
- Cellulitis
- Burns
- Severe dermatitis at site
- Vasculitis
- Contralateral pneumothorax or hemothorax

- Inability of patient to tolerate ipsilateral pneumothorax
- Indwelling vascular hardware
- Injury proximal to the insertion site.

Again in all these situations ultrasound guidance offers substantial cumulative benefits in terms of safety and success.

EQUIPMENT SPECIFICATIONS

For Ultrasound

- *Transducer:* linear array transducers of frequencies between 7.5 and 12 MHz are generally preferred. Small-footprint probes are used in pediatric patients or in areas where space is limited, such as near the clavicle.
- Color Doppler imaging and pulse wave Doppler should be used for identifying flow in vascular structures and differentiating arteries from veins.
- Sterile probe covers or sterile gloves can be used to cover probe.
- Echogenic needle tips for access may improve sonographic visibility.

Other Equipments

Common central venous lines include:
Set of central venous line
- Single lumen: 16, 18, or 20 gauge; 8, 12, or 15 cm
- Double lumen: 18/18 gauge, 7.5 F; 15, 20, 25 cm
- Triple lumen: 18/18/16 gauge; 7 F; 15, 20, 25 cm
- Sterile gown, gloves, mask and hair cover
- Local anesthetic, syringe, small gauge needle
- Sterile antiseptic solution
- Finder needle (22 gauge)
- Introducer needle (16 or 18 gauge)

- Guidewire
- No. 11 blade scalpel
- Vein dilator
- Full sterile sheet and sterile towels
- Sterile normal saline flushes, 10 mL each
- IV tubing, flushes, syringe
- Central venous catheter
- 3-0 silk suture with needle and needle holder
- Antibacterial patch
- Sterile gauze pads and sterile dressing

GENERAL PROTOCOL FOR CENTRAL LINE PLACEMENT

Here are the few protocols which we should follow while cannulatig central vein.

Preparations for CV Placement

- Written informed consent and indications for procedure
- Perform the procedure in an environment that permits use of aseptic techniques
- A standardized equipment set should be available for central venous access
- Make a checklist and fix protocol should be used for placement and maintenance of central venous catheters
- An assistant should be used during placement of a central venous catheter.

Precautions to Prevent Complications

Infectious Complications

Following measures should be taken to prevent infectious complications associated with central venous access:

- Aseptic techniques
- Use of intravenous antibiotic prophylaxis
- Use coated or impregnated catheters
- Proper selection of catheter insertion site
- Catheter fixation method
- Proper dressings at insertion site.

Aseptic preparation: In preparation for the placement of central venous catheters always use full aseptic techniques including proper hand washing along with maximal barrier precautions, which reduces catheters-related infections (e.g. sterile gowns, sterile gloves, caps, masks covering both mouth and nose, and full-body patient drapes).

Use of intravenous antibiotic prophylaxis: It is recommended that for immunocompromised patients and high-risk neonates intravenous antibiotic prophylaxis should be given prior to procedure, Intravenous antibiotic prophylaxis should not be administered routinely.

Antiseptic solution: A chlorhexidine-containing solution should be used for skin preparation. If there is a contraindication to chlorhexidine, povidone-iodine or alcohol may be used. Catheter tip colonization reduces with povidone iodine alone.

Use of catheters containing antimicrobial agents: Catheters coated with antibiotics or a combination of chlorhexidine and silver sulfadiazine are available which should be used for selected patients based on infectious risk, cost and anticipated duration of catheter use, which reduces catheter colonization.

Selection of catheter insertion site: Catheter insertion site selection should be based on clinical need. An insertion site should be selected that is not contaminated or potentially contaminated (e.g. burned or infected skin, inguinal area, adjacent to tracheostomy or open surgical wound). In adults, selection of an upper body insertion site should be considered to minimize the risk of infection. Femoral insertion site is associated with higher levels of catheter colonization compared to IJV and subclavian.

Catheter fixation technique: The use of sutures is the preferred catheter fixation technique to minimize catheter-related infection, or staples and tape can also be used.

Dressings at insertion site: Transparent bio-occlusive dressings should be used to protect the site of central venous catheter insertion from infection.

Catheter maintenance:
- Catheters should be removed promptly when no longer deemed clinically necessary. The catheter insertion site should be inspected daily for signs of infection.
- Catheter should be changed or removed when catheter insertion site infection is suspected.
- When a catheter related infection is suspected, replacing the catheter using a new insertion site is preferable to changing the catheter over a guidewire.

Prevention of Mechanical Trauma or Injury

Following measures should be taken to prevent mechanical trauma or injury associated with central venous access:
- Select proper catheter insertion site
- Proper positioning of the patient for needle insertion and catheter placement
- Monitoring for needle, guidewire and catheter placement.

Selection of catheter insertion site: The femoral site had a higher frequency of thrombotic complications in adult patients. Internal jugular insertion site is preferred to minimize catheter cannulation-related risk of injury or trauma. Arterial puncture, hematoma, pneumothorax, hemothorax, arrhythmias are common with internal jugular and subclvian insertion.

Positioning of the patient for needle insertion and catheter placement: When clinically appropriate and feasible, central venous access in the neck or chest should be performed with the patient in the Trendelenburg position in adults , in which the diameter of the internal jugular vein increases and there are reduced chances of air embolism, particularly in dehydrated patients.

Needle insertion and catheter placement: Routinely we prefer the smallest size catheter appropriate for the clinical situation. The Seldinger technique that is catheter over-the-needle provides more stable venous access.

Guidance and confirmation of needle and catheter placement: Nowadays ultrasound is the best way for needle and catheter placement. This can be done using static (prepuncture vessel localization) or dynamic (real time vessel localization) method. Other methods include: (1) manometry, (2) continuous electrocardiography, (3) chest radiography.

Continuous electrocardiography is effective in identifying proper catheter tip placement and chest radiograph should be performed to confirm the location of the catheter tip as soon after catheterization as clinically appropriate.

Management of Arterial Trauma or Injury due to Central Venous Catheterization

When accidental cannulation of an arterial vessel occurs, the dilator or catheter should be left in place and a general surgeon, a vascular surgeon, or an interventional radiologist should be immediately consulted regarding surgical or nonsurgical catheter removal for adults.

Once the injury has been evaluated and a treatment plan has been executed, the anesthesiologist and surgeon should consider relative risks and benefits of proceeding with the elective surgery *versus* deferring surgery to allow for a period of patient observation.

GENERAL CONSIDERATION FOR ULTRASOUND-GUIDED VASCULAR ACCESS

As with all procedures, always take proper history and perform physical examination to determine the appropriate procedure and anatomic site. Evaluate for known anatomic issues, prior procedures, and the potential for complications (particularly the presence of an underlying coagulopathy). For central venous access, written informed consent should generally be obtained unless the procedure is emergent.

Plane of Visualization (Fig. 1)

Short-axis (Out-of-Plane) Versus Long-Axis (In-Plane) Visualization

There are two basic sonographic views used to obtain image of vessels: short axis or long axis.

Using basic B-mode imaging, the plane of the ultrasound image may be oriented relative to the vessel in the short (out-of-plane) or long (in-plane) axis. In a short-axis view, the image plane is perpendicular to the course of the vessel, so the needle should be inserted from center of the vein (Fig. 2), so needle is 'out-of-plane'. To obtain this image, simply follow the orientation rule: probe marker toward the left of the person performing procedure, and align the marker from the probe with the indicator in the display. The vessel will appear as an

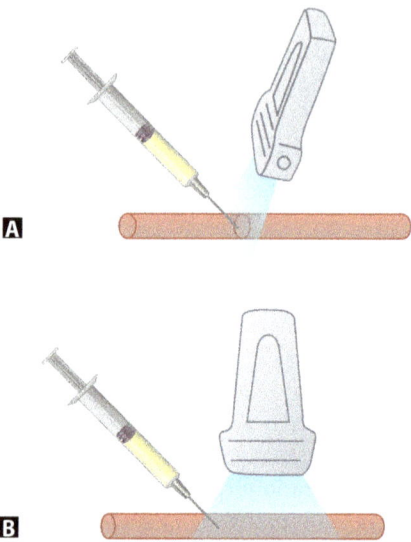

Figs 1A and B: (A) Out-of-plane approach short axis view; (B) In-plane approach

anechoic circle on the screen with the needle visualized as a hyperechoic point in cross section. In a long-axis view, the image plane will be seen parallel to the course of the vessel (needle is "in-plane")(Fig. 3).

In long-axis view we have advantage of assessing the anterior and posterior walls of the vein being cannulated, thus avoiding double puncturing of the vessel, and also we can visualize entire needle shaft and tip, but the disadvantage is that it may be more difficult to keep the plane of the ultrasound in line with the vessel as the plane of the image may "slip off" to the side of the plane of the needle and/or the center of the vessel.

The long-axis approach may be easier and more appropriate to use in larger vessels such as central veins when knowing the tip location is crucial, although with experience and care, the short-axis approach is adequate

Ultrasound-guided Central Venous Access

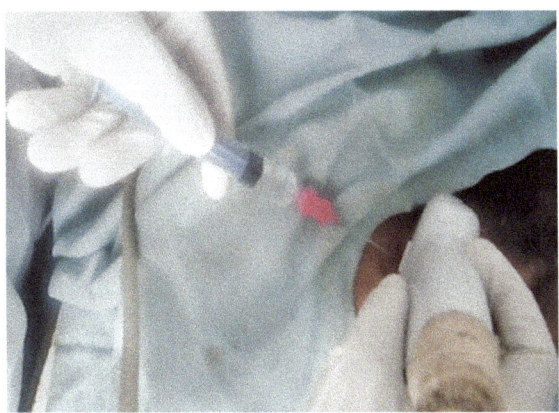

Fig. 2: Probe position for out-of-plane approach

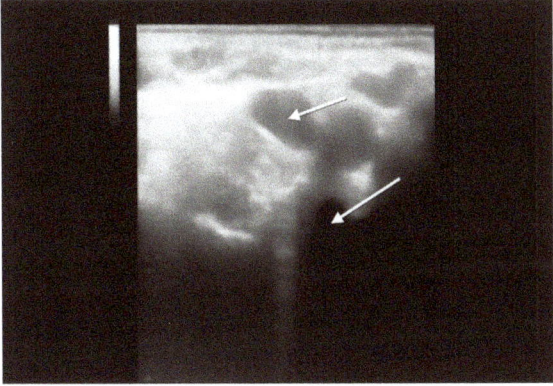

Fig. 3: US image of out-of-plane approach: anechoic vein is seen with only the tip of needle. Arrows show the tip of the needle with ring down artifact

and sufficient to follow the needle tip location. It may be helpful to start a procedure with a short-axis view to ensure that the needle is centered over the middle of the vessel and then rotate the probe to a long-axis (in-plane view) as the needle is advanced (Fig. 4).

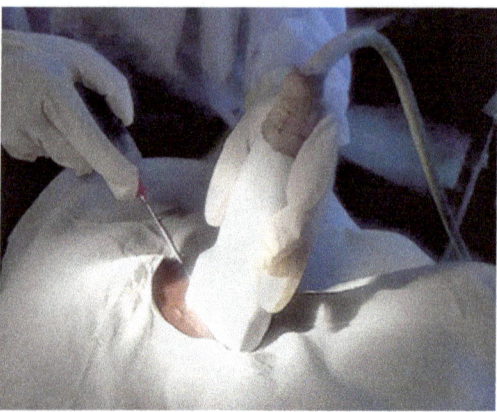

Fig. 4: Probe position for in-plane approach

Short-axis (out-of-plane)	Long-axis (in-plane)
Image plane is perpendicular to the course of the vessel and to the needle (needle is "out-of-plane"). The vessel should appear as an anechoic circle on the screen with the needle visualized as a hyperechoic point in cross section.	The image plane is parallel to the course of the vessel (needle is "in-plane"). The image should show the course of the vessel across the screen and the shaft and point of the needle as it is advanced.
The short-axis view allows the needle approach to be over the center of the vein. However, care must be taken to "fan" the plane of the image along the needle as it advances to track the tip and avoid underestimating the depth of the tip.	The long-axis view has the advantage of allowing visualization of the entire needle shaft and tip, it may be more difficult to keep the plane of the ultrasound in line with the vessel as the plane of the image may "slip off" to the side of the plane of the needle and/or center of the vessel (Fig. 5).
It may be helpful to start a procedure with a short-axis view to ensure that the needle is centered over the middle of the vessel.	The long-axis approach may be easier and more appropriate to use in larger vessels such as central veins when knowing the tip location is crucial.

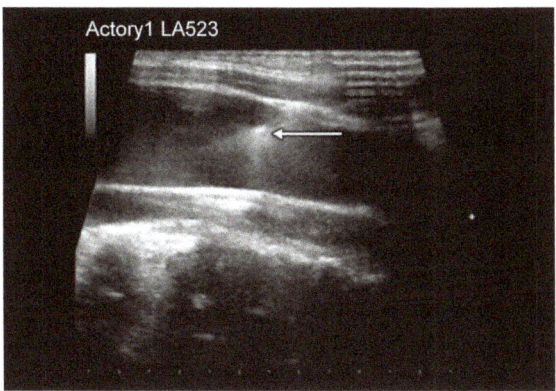

Fig. 5: Ultrasound image: Whole vein with needle is seen. Arrow shows the vein with shaft and point of the needle

Differentiating Arteries from Veins

Ultrasound Characteristics of Arterial and Venous Flow

In ultrasound first we should know the exact anatomical landmarks to start with scanning. Both arteries and veins appear anechoic on ultrasound. The Doppler capability should be used to distinguish hypoechoic structures as vascular vs. non-vascular before introducing needles to the field.

In color Doppler mode, any blood flow towards the transducer will be red on screen, and flow away from the transducer will be blue on screen. For vascular access, arteries and veins are conventionally approached from their anticipated anatomical relationships with surface landmarks. This principle remains relatively unchanged in the ultrasound-guided approach.

If color signal is not seen from a suspected blood vessel, the structure being assessed may not be vascular, may not have any flow within it (as is the case with a thrombosed vessel), or the transducer may be oriented perpendicular to the flow, and is therefore not being detected.

Another method for assessment is Color Power Doppler. Color power Doppler can detect even low flow.

In short,
- Arteries and veins appear same on a gray scale ultrasound image
- Both have an anechoic (black) lumen
  The arteries have thicker walls that are seen more hyperechoic (brighter) than the walls of veins (Fig. 6)
- Arteries are less compressible than veins, but the ability to compress venous walls with relatively minimal pressure is a useful way to distinguish a vein from an artery
- Peripheral vessels are more easily compressible than central vessels, but central vessels may be fairly easily compressed in a hypotensive patient. A noncompressible venous lumen indicates a thrombus

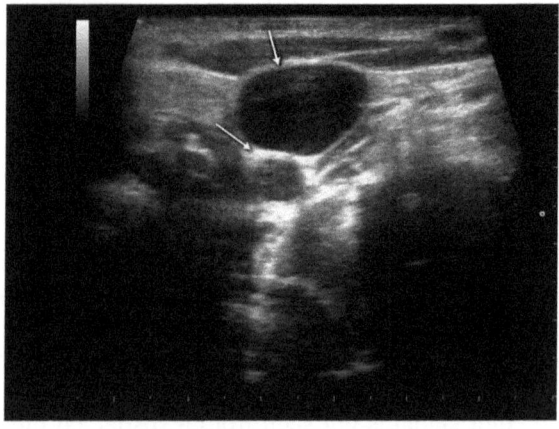

Fig. 6: Short arrow shows venous wall which is thin, long arrow shows thick wall which is arterial wall

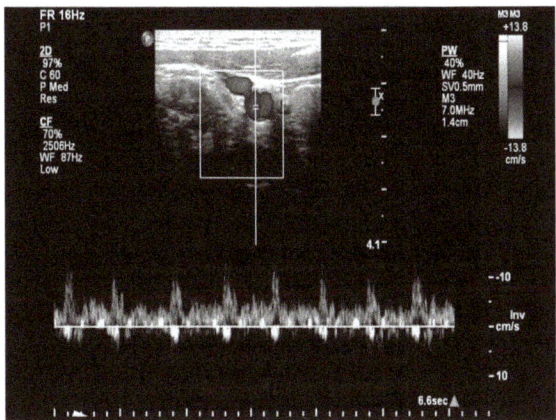

Fig. 7: Pulse wave Doppler shows artery is pulsatile (Blue). In US it is not necessary that artey is seen red and vein blue, it depends on the flow of the vessel. Blue away from the transducer and red towards the transducer

- Doppler imaging should be used to identify blood flow and to help differentiate arterial from venous flow (Fig. 7).

Static Versus Dynamic Ultrasound Guidance

There are two ways by which we can perform the procedure:

Static Method

Here we do prescanning to determine the vessel location and patency, assess surrounding structures, and mark the location to provide optimum placement for needle introduction. Once we localize the vessel we put mark over there, remove the probe and perform the procedure without real-time ultrasound. The static approach has advantages over a completely landmark-guided procedure.

Dynamic Approach

In dynamic approach after scanning we perform the procedure under real-time ultrasound guidance. Here we can visualize the needle tip placement as well as catheter. It has been shown to be superior to the static approach in most situations. It is used for the internal jugular vein and femoral veins, and is also, but less commonly, used for the subclavian vein.

One-person Versus Two-person Technique

In a one-person dynamic approach, the person performing the procedure holds the needle with one hand while directing the ultrasound probe in the other hand. A one-person dynamic approach requires more experience and it is preferred by most advanced practitioners, as it allows for real-time hand-eye coordination.

In two-person approach one person localizes the vein and other person performs the procedure. This provides the potential advantage of allowing the person performing the procedure to use two hands for the procedure itself and does not require the dual hand-eye coordination of directing the ultrasound transducer as well as performing the procedure.

Site Selection and Preparation

The choice of site depends on factors such as vessel size, depth, course, surrounding structures, and adjacent pathology (such as overlying cellulitis). Assess the vessel for patency, course, and other anatomic issues such as vein valves.

For long-term central access, the IJV and subclavian vein are preferred over femoral vein because of high infection rates. But in trauma and shock patients femoral vein is easily accessible and becomes a good choice in such situations.

Ultrasound-guided Central Venous Access

Location	Advantages	Disadvantages
IJV	• Bleeding can be recognized and controlled • Malposition is rare • Less risk of pneumothorax	• Risk of carotid artery puncture • PTX possible
Subclavian	Most comfortable for conscious patients	• Highest risk of PTX Should not do on intubated patients • Should not be done if <2 years • Vein is non-compressible
Femoral	• Easy to find vein • No risk of pneumothorax • Preferred site for emergencies and CPR • Fewer bad complications	• Highest risk of infection • Risk of DVT • Not good for ambulatory patients

Abbreviations: IJV, Internal jugular vein; PTX, pentoxifylline; DVT, deep vein thrombosis

- Once a site has been chosen, the site and ultrasound equipment should be prepared for the procedure, and preprocedural local anesthesia may be applied and/or injected.
- After adequate anesthesia, prepare the chosen site for central venous or arterial access using maximal sterile barrier precautions.
- Ultrasound probe requires additional sterile cover. The gel must be placed both inside and outside the sheath, with sterile gel used on the outside. Avoid air bubbles between the face of the probe and the inner surface of the sterile sheath, as this will lead to suboptimal visualization.

ULTRASOUND-GUIDED VASCULAR ACCESS LINE PLACEMENT

There are three major sites for accomplishing CVC access: (1) Internal jugular vein, (2) subclavian and (3) femoral.

The internal jugular and femoral veins are easy to perform under ultrasound guidance while subclavian vein may be more challenging to visualize with ultrasound due to interference from the clavicle. Access to the subclavian vein via the axillary vein or via a supraclavicular approach may be more amenable to ultrasound.

A pre-procedure scan should be performed before sterile precautions are taken precautions are taken to identify thrombi, occlusion and unfavorable anatomy.

The anatomy of each site as well as the advantages, disadvantages, and special considerations for each are discussed below.

Internal Jugular Vein

Anatomy (Fig. 8)

On both sides and at the base of the brain, the *inferior petrosal sinus* and the *sigmoid sinus join* to form the internal jugular vein. The internal jugular vein begins in the posterior compartment of the *jugular foramen*, at the base of the *skull*. Then IJ vein exits the skull through the jugular foramen just anteromedial to the mastoid process, then it runs down the side of the neck in a vertical direction, being at one end lateral to the *internal carotid artery*, and then lateral to the common carotid, and at the root of the neck, it unites with the *subclavian vein* to form the *brachiocephalic vein* (innominate vein).

It increases in diameter as it descends, making it easier to cannulate below the cricoid cartilage. The

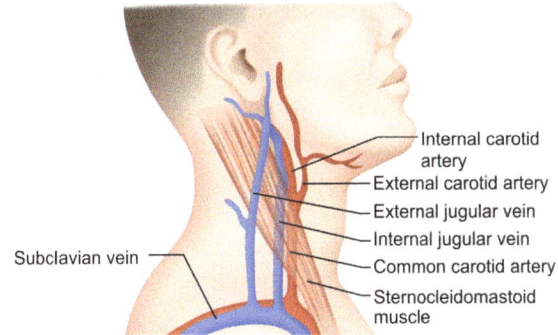

Fig. 8: Anatomy of internal jugular, subclavian and adjacent vessels

apex of the right lung is also lower than the apex of the left lung, slightly decreasing the risk of pneumothorax compared with the left side.

As the site of IJ vein is easily accessible it makes it collapsible and compressible, and thus it is a more preferred site to the subclavian, especially in anticoagulated patients. The IJ vein can be accessed by several different approaches: anterior, central, and posterior.

Anterior: Medial to the sternocleidomastoid (SCM) muscle at the level of the thyroid cartilage to the skin.

Posterior: 1 cm superior to where the EJ crosses the SCM lateral edge or one-third of the way from clavicle to mastoid process.

Central: Superior apex of 2 heads of the SCM.

Special Considerations, Advantages, and Disadvantages

Relative contraindications for internal jugular vein cannulation

Interval jugular vein cannulation should be avoided in cervical spine fractures, penetrating neck injury, and left bundle branch block, because central venous catheter placement is a possible trigger for complete heart block. Also, as carotid artery lies medial to the IJV carotid artery puncture is a possible complication. If there is accidental arterial puncture, remove the needle and apply pressure for a minimum of 5 minutes (double if coagulopathy is present). Do not attempt IJ cannulation on the other side. If the catheter is placed in the carotid artery, do not remove the catheter and consult vascular surgeon.

Ultrasound is particularly useful in patients on mechanical ventilator for success as well as to decrease mechanical and infectious complications, particularly in hypovolemic patients.

Advantages of the IJ vein include the direct course to right atrium for hemodialysis catheters and transvenous pacers.

Disadvantages include possible carotid artery puncture and patient preference.

TECHNIQUE FOR INTERNAL JUGULAR VEIN CANNULATION

Positioning: For IJV and SV access, patients should be placed in a slightly *Trendelenburg position*. The head should be in a neutral position (maximum head rotation of 30–45°).

Technique for IJV Cannulation

Performing the Procedure

- To insert a central venous catheter, prepare a sterile field that includes the necessary equipment. Always gown, prep, and drape in a sterile manner. Open the central venous catheter kit in a sterile manner, or

have an assistant prepare the equipment in a sterile manner. Prepare the central venous catheter by flushing all ports and lumens with sterile saline
- The ultrasound system should be placed parallel to the patient on the same side as the procedure to align anatomic landmarks with the image display
- Place a sterile sheath with transducer gel inside the sheath and sterile gel outside the sheath on the transducer
  Using the linear probe in the transverse plane, locate the vein and corresponding artery. Place the transducer according to anatomic site of the vessel and look for the anatomic variations, width and depth of vessel, and sign of venous thrombosis
- The vein will be compressible and thin walled compared with the artey. Center the vein in the image and estimate the depth. Needle placement can be performed in either of the 2 views discussed earlier: short- or long-axis view
- Local anesthesia should be given to patient to reduce pain and movement of the patient while performing the procedure. Use injection lidocaine and inject around the trajectory of the needle, including muscles and subcutaneous tissue
- Stabilize transducer with the sterile probe cover with one hand and then insert 18-gauge needle with the dominant hand under real guidance, through the anterior wall of the vein and into the lumen.

To assess trajectory and distance of the needle to puncture the vessel, we use the principles of the Pythagoras theorem (Fig. 9) for right-angled triangles. If the vessel to cannulate is seen 1 cm deep, puncture the skin 1 cm away from the transducer at a 45 angle to create an isosceles triangle. Here the needle should be inserted up to the distance of 1.4 cm to reach the top of the vessel (Pythagoras theorem = $a^2 + b^2 = c^2$).

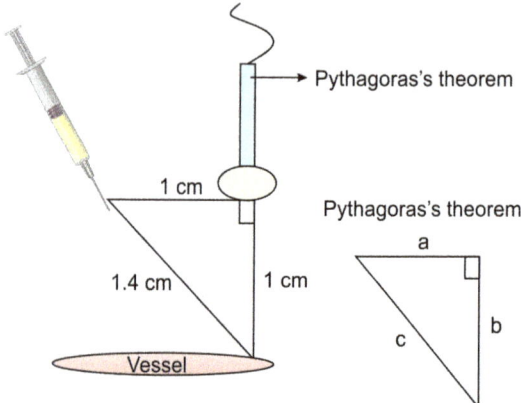

Fig. 9: Pythagoras's theorem

- In the short-axis approach, transducer should be placed on the neck and trace the internal jugular vein from above downwards (**apex of the triangle to base of the triangle in which the IJV lies**). Now move the transducer in such a way that image of the vessel should be seen in the center of the ultrasound screen, and this will serve as landmark for needle insertion.
  - Insert the needle from the center of the probe, when needle reaches the vein it will create **bright echo** with ring-down artifact on the screen, then aspirate the blood.
  - Now insert the guidewire, it will be seen in the center (movement will be seen)
- For the long-axis approach (In Plane method): First locate the vein in short axis view, then rotate the transducer at 90°, so the entire image of IJV can be seen parallel to the probe, it is important to keep the hand stable to place the transducer parallel to the vessel.

Ultrasound-guided Central Venous Access

- Now insert the needle from the marker side, when needle reaches the vein we can visualize whole needle in the vein (Fig. 10)
- Then aspirate the blood
- Insert the guidewire, it will be seen in the center. Here movement will be seen.

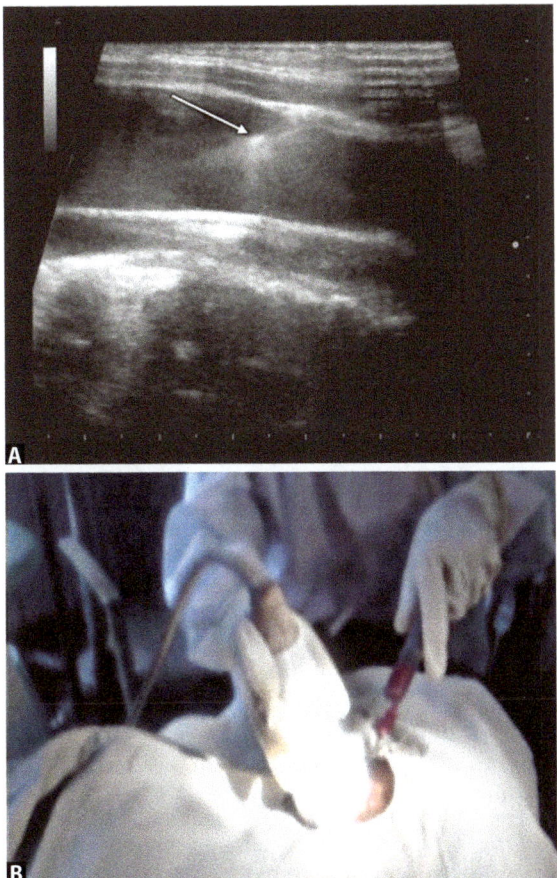

Figs 10A and B: Arrow shows needle tip with shaft

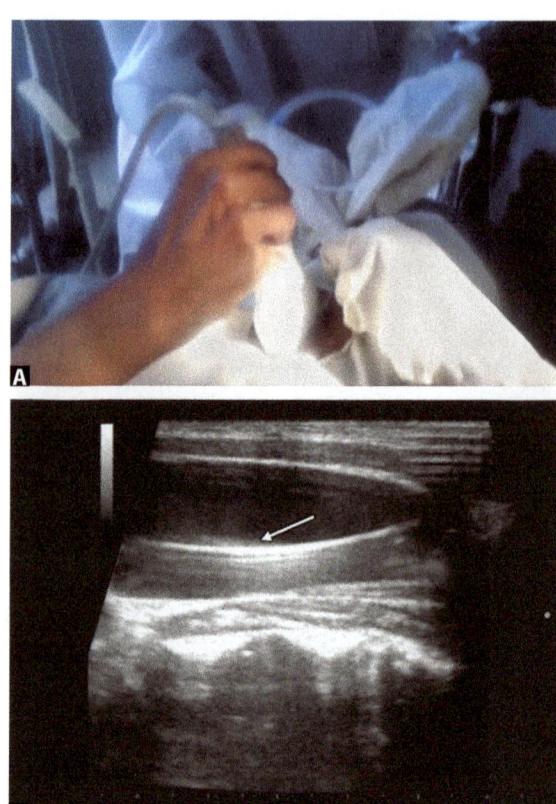

Figs 11A and B: Arrow shows guidewire

Placement of the guidewire, dilator, and line may then proceed. Direct visualization of the guidewire/dilator within the vein can ensure proper placement (Figs 11 to 13). Sterile technique should be maintained at all times.

Evaluate: Ultrasound can be used to confirm the guidewire within the lumen before dilating the vessel. The catheter appears as a linear "white" shadow that is best appreciated in the longitudinal ultrasound view.

Ultrasound-guided Central Venous Access

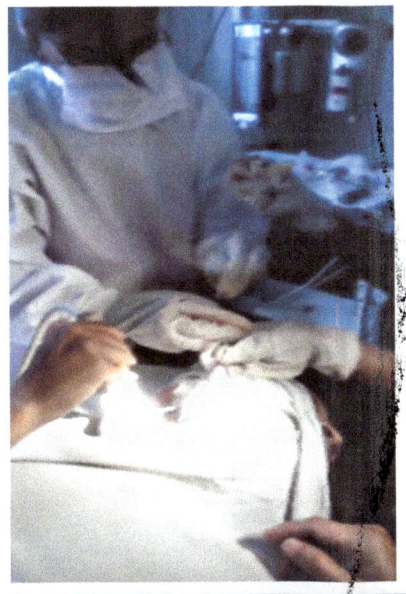

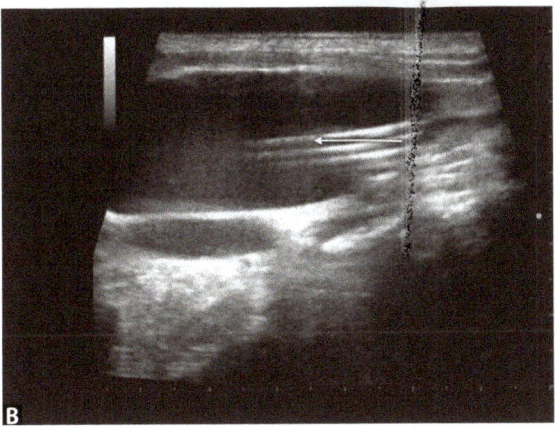

Figs 12A and B: Shows catheter over guidewire.
Arrow shows all three layers of catheter with guidewire

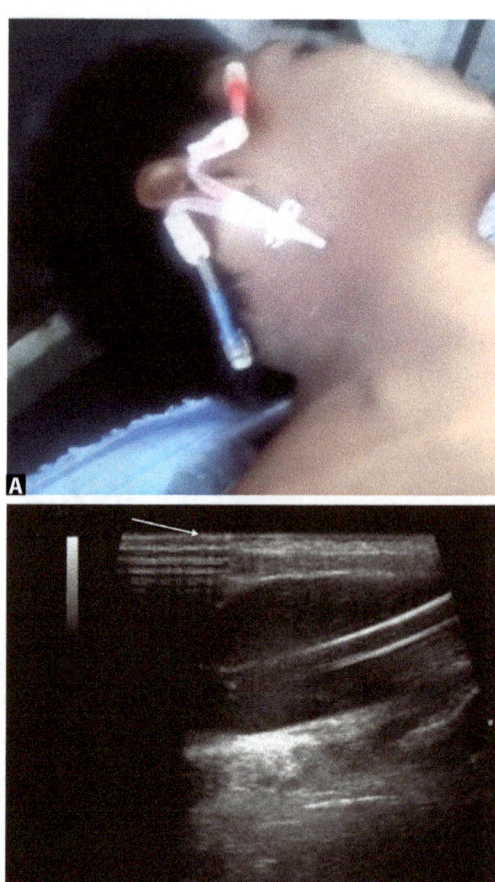

Figs 13A and B: Arrow shows catheter after removal of guidewire

IMPORTANT FACTS
(Problems Arising During Cannulation and Their Solution)

- Stabilization of the transducer may be difficult so, it is recommended to become familiar with the short-axis approach before the long axis. Whichever approach is being used introduce the needle at a 45 to 60 angle aiming toward the probe marker, and follow the trajectory of the needle as it goes into the anterior wall of the vessel. Once vessel is punctured remove the ultrasound probe proceed with the standard Seldinger technique

- The image on the ultrasound monitor is a two-dimensional representation of three-dimensional structures
- The center of the ultrasound image on the monitor corresponds to the center of the ultrasound probe, which is important for needle insertion
- On the geometrical basis we should do skin puncture at a 45-degree angle a distance from the probe that is equal to the depth of the vessel. That means if the vessel is localized 1 cm below the skin surface, the ideal skin puncture should be done at 1 cm from the ultrasound probe at a 45-degree angle
- Most of needles are sonolucent, so may not be visible in ultrasound and vessel puncture can be confirmed by vessel tenting from needle pressure and a small amount of flash artifact from the needle tip
- There are commercially available needles coated in a sonographically opaque material that allow greater visibility of the needle.

Subclavian Vein

Each subclavian vein is a continuation of the axillary vein and runs from the outer border of the first rib to the medial border of anterior scalene muscle. From here it joins with the internal jugular vein to form the brachicephalic vein (also known as "innominate vein"). The subclavian vein follows the subclavian artery and is separated from the subclavian artery by the insertion of anterior scalene. Thus, the subclavian vein lies anterior to the anterior scalene while the subclavian artery lies posterior to the anterior scalene (and anterior to the middle scalene).

The subclavian vein is accessed by either an infraclavicular or supraclavicular approach. There are high success rate and less-frequent catheter malpositioning than the infraclavicular approach. Again it depends on the operator's experience.

Special Considerations, Advantages and Disadvantages

Complication rate is low with subclavian venous cannulation.

Relative contraindications include chest wall deformities, clavicle fractures, first or second rib fractures, or clavicle surgery on same side.

Advantages of subclavian venous access include a high degree of patient tolerance, a similarly low complication rate to the IJ, and the ease of insertion.

Disadvantages include risk of subclavian artery puncture (a noncompressible site) and an increased risk of pneumothorax.

TECHNIQUE FOR SUBCLAVIAN VEIN

Usually out of plane method is used to cannulate Subclavian vein. There are two approaches: Supraclavicular and Infraclavicular.

Supraclavicular Approach

Supraclavicular approach has higher success rate and less catheter malpositioning than infraclavicular approach, but chances of Aorta puncture are more as arch of aorta lies near to it, So we have to be very careful while cannulating subclavian vein through supraclavicular approach. Trace the probe from apex of the triangle formed by meeting point of two sternocleidomastoid

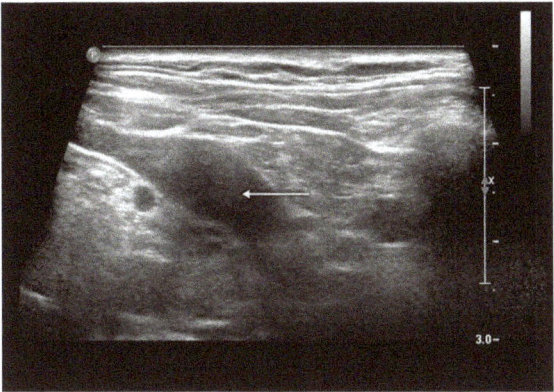

Fig. 14: Arrow shows brachicephalic vein as seen in supraclavicular approach

muscle, bring the probe up to the base of triangle then tilt probe downwards, here IJV meets with the subclavian vein to form a brachiocephalic vein (Fig. 14). This is the largest vein formed, the advantage is that it can be easily cannulated even in shock and cardiac arrest patients. Insert the needle from center of the probe, Rest of the procedure is same as IJV.

Infraclavicular Approach

The infraclavicular approach is little difficult by US guidance because here the subclavian vein lies beneath the clavicle. In this approach, the probe is placed vertically on the mid-clavicle, a big subclavian vein can be seen (Fig. 15). Bring the image by moving the probe in the center of the screen, insert the needle from center of the probe. Rest of the procedure is same as IJV cannulation.

- **Femoral vein (Fig. 16):** The **femoral vein** accompanies the femoral artery in the femoral sheath. It begins at the adductor canal as a continuation of the popliteal vein. It ends at the inferior margin of the inguinal ligament, where it becomes the external iliac vein.

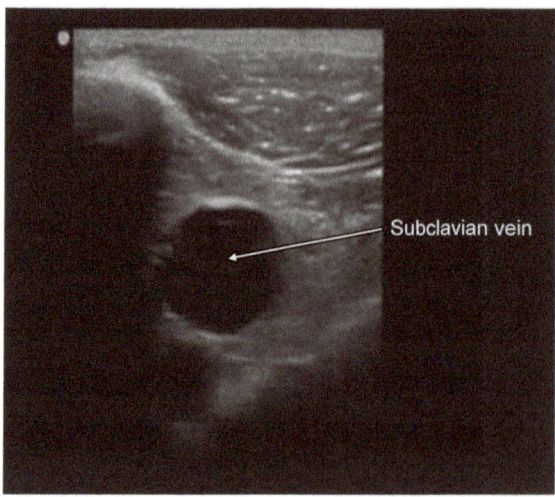

Fig. 15: Subclavian vein as seen in infraclavicular approach

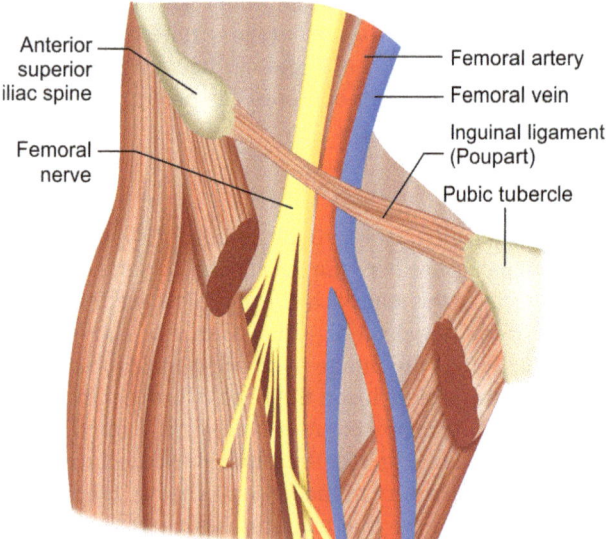

Fig. 16: Femoral vein anatomy

Ultrasound-guided Central Venous Access

- The location of the femoral vein makes it the largest and easiest site for central venous access.

It is encased in the femoral sheath with the femoral artery, nerve, and lymphatics. The anatomy of the vessels can be described with a simple mnemonic: NAVEL.

From lateral to medial, the structures in the sheath are femoral nerve, femoral artery, femoral vein, empty space, lymphatics (Fig. 17).

Special Considerations, Advantages and Disadvantages

- Femoral vein should be avoided if there is significant trauma to the lower extremity or deep venous thrombosis on same side.
- Avoid femoral cannulation in case of abdominal trauma which may interrupt the inferior vena cava. Blood return below the diaphragm during cardiopulmonary resuscitation may be reduced.
- The femoral vein is the largest and easiest central vein to access; but, there is a higher rate of venous thrombosis and line infection at this site. Femoral vein cannulation should be used for CVP monitoring

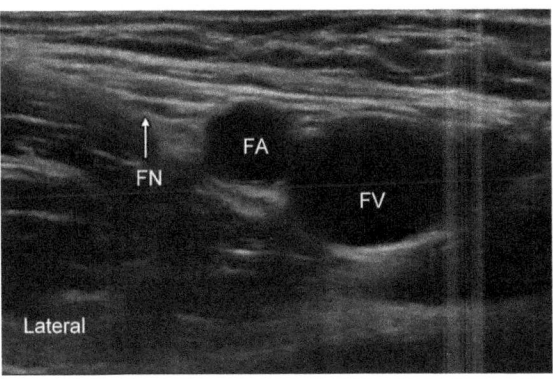

Fig. 17: Sonoanatomy of femoral vein

when the more common jugular and subclavian sites are not accessible, as in patients with burns, trauma, or surgical procedures that involve the head, neck, and upper thorax.
- Complications of central venous catheterization like pneumothorax and carotid or subclavian arterial injury can be avoided when femoral vein is cannulated.
- Femoral venipuncture should be performed below the inguinal ligament just medial to the palpated femoral arterial pulse in a manner similar to that used for femoral arterial cannulation. Either a long (40-70 cm) catheter should be used, using ECG guidance, in the inferior vena cava close to the cavoatrial junction, or a shorter (15-20 cm) catheter should be inserted from the femoral vein into the common iliac vein. Both techniques can provide intra-abdominal venous pressure measurements that agree closely with simultaneously obtained superior vena caval CVPs when these pressures are measured in mechanically ventilated, critically ill adults.
- Potential disadvantages of the femoral venous route include increased risks of thromboembolic and infectious complications, although the magnitude of these risks has not been established. In addition, femoral arterial or venous injury during attempted cannulation may result in intra-abdominal hemorrhage.

TECHNIQUE FOR FEMORAL VEIN CANNULATION

- **Position of the patient:** As femoral vein lies deep to the artery chances of arterial puncture are high so patient should be given supine position with leg slightly externally rotated (frog leg position).

- Femoral vein can be cannulated by both in plane and out of plane approach. The probe position is decided by palpating the femoral artery. Rest of the method is same as in other central veins.

ALTERNATIVE CENTRAL VENOUS CANNULATION SITES

Left Internal Jugular Vein

In conditions where right internal jugular vein cannulation cannot be performed, e.g. burns, sepsis at local site, left interal jugular vein should be cannulated.

The disadvantages are:
- The cupola of the pleura is higher on the left than on the right, theoretically increasing the risk of pneumothorax.
- The thoracic duct may be injured during venipuncture, because it enters the venous system at the junction of the left internal jugular and subclavian veins.
- The left internal jugular vein is often smaller than the right and demonstrates a greater degree of overlap of the adjacent carotid artery during head rotation.
- Catheters inserted from the left side of the patient must traverse the innominate (i.e. left brachiocephalic) vein and enter the superior vena cava perpendicularly, and their distal tips may impinge on the right lateral wall of the superior vena cava, thereby increasing the risk of vascular injury (This anatomic disadvantage pertains to all left-sided catheterization sites and highlights the need for radiographic confirmation of proper catheter location).
- Clinicians usually cannulate the left internal jugular vein much less often than the right, it is not surprising that cannulation of the left internal jugular vein is

more difficult, more time-consuming, and associated with more complications than right internal jugular cannulation.

External Jugular Vein

Both the right and left external jugular veins provide a safe alternative to internal jugular or subclavian vein cannulation.

Advantages of external jugular vein cannulation:

- The external jugular veins are superficial structures, they allow central venous cannulation with essentially no risk of pneumothorax or unintended arterial puncture.
- In most instances, it is best to use an 18-gauge catheter, rather than the thin-wall needle, to introduce the guidewire because of the tortuous course of the external jugular vein and the frequent need to manipulate the guidewire repeatedly to guide it into the superior vena cava.
- A J-tip guidewire should always be used, because it may be advanced under the clavicle into the central circulation more successfully than a straight-tip wire.
- When the guidewire does not advance as desired and appears to be moving peripherally into the subclavian vein, central venous passage may be facilitated by abducting the ipsilateral shoulder beyond 90 degrees prior to advancing the wire. Alternatively, the patient's ipsilateral arm is placed at the side, and an assistant applies mild caudad traction on the shoulder to straighten the course of the external jugular vein while the wire is advanced.
- Essentially the only factors that preclude use of the external jugular veins for CVP monitoring are an inability to visualize and cannulate the vessel in the neck and to advance a catheter into the central

circulation. Unfortunately, these problems occur in approximately 20% of patients, thus limiting more widespread application of this technique.

DOCUMENTATION

Documentation is must for all procedures. Here we get the added advantage of ultrasound guidance, so detail record of patient, procedural image should be preserved.

BIBLIOGRAPHY

1. Armstrong PJ, Sutherland R, Scott DH. The effect of position and different manoeuvres on the internal jugular vein diameter size. Acta Anaesth Scand. 1994;38:229-31.
2. Ault MJ, Rosen BT, Ault BW. Inadvertent carotid artery cannulation during ultrasound guided central venous catheterization. Ann Emerg Med. 2006;49:721.
3. Bach A, Schmidt H, Bttiger B, Schreiber B, Bhrer H, Motsch J, et al. Retention of antibacterial activity and bacterial colonization of antiseptic-bonded central venous catheters. J Antimicrob Chemother. 1996;37:315-22.
4. Bellazzini MA, Rankin PM, Gangnon RE, Bjoernsen LP. Ultrasound validation of maneuvers to increase internal jugular vein cross-sectional area and decrease compressibility. Am J Emerg Med. 2009;27:454-9.
5. Berenholtz SM, Pronovost PJ, Lipsett PA, Hobson D, Earsing K, Farley JE. Eliminating catheter-related bloodstream infections in the intensive care unit. Crit Care Med. 2004;32:2014-20.
6. Blaivas M, Adhikari S. An unseen danger: frequency of posterior vessel wall penetration by needles during attempts to place internal jugular vein central catheters using ultrasound guidance. Crit Care Med. 2009;37:2345-9.
7. Brun-Buisson C, Doyon F, Sollet JP, Cochard JF, Cohen Y, Nitenberg G. Prevention of intravascular catheter-related infection with newer chlorhexidine-silver

sulfadiazinecoated catheters: A randomized controlled trial. Intensive Care Med. 2004;30:837-43.
8. Ciresi DL, Albrecht RM, Volkers PA, Scholten DJ. Failure of antiseptic bonding to prevent central venous catheter-related infection and sepsis. Am Surg. 1996;62:641-6.
9. Collignon P, Soni N, Pearson I, Sorrell T, Woods P. Sepsis associated with central vein catheters in critically ill patients. Intensive Care Med. 1988;14:227-31.
10. Critical skills and Procedures in Emergency Medicine: Vascular Access skills and procedures : Gemma C. Lewis, Stephanie A. Crapo, Jefferson G. Wiliams. 2013.
11. Cummins RO. Advanced cardiac life support. Dallas (TX): American Heart Association; 1994;1-13.
12. Denys BG, Uretsky BF. Anatomical variations of internal jugular vein location: impact on central venous access. Crit Care Med. 1991;19:1516.
13. Deshpande KS, Hatem C, Ulrich H, et al. The incidence of infectious complications of central venous catheters at the subclavian, internal jugular, and femoral sites in an intensive care unit population. Crit Care Med. 2005; 33(1):13-20.
14. Eisenhauer ED, Derveloy RJ, Hastings PR. Prospective evaluation of central venous pressure (CVP) catheters in a large city-county hospital. Ann Surg. 1982;196:560.
15. Eissa NT, Kvetan V. Guide wire as a cause of complete heart block in patients with preexisting left bundle branch block. Anesthesiology. 1990;73:772-4.
16. Feldman R. Central venous access. In: Reichman EF, Simon RR, (Eds). Emergency medicine procedures. New York: McGraw-Hill; 2004; 314-37.
17. Gil RT, Kruse JA, Thill-Baharozian MC, Carlson RW. Triple vs single-lumen central venous catheters: A prospective study in a critically ill population. Arch Intern Med. 1989; 149:1139-43.
18. Gowardman JR, Robertson IK, Parkes S, Rickard CM. Influence of insertion site on central venous catheter colonization and bloodstream infection rates. Intensive Care Med. 2008;34:1038-45.

19. Guilbert MC, Elkouri S, Bracco D, Corriveau MM, Beaudoin N, Dubois MJ, et al. Arterial trauma during central venous catheter insertion: Case series, review and proposed algorithm. J Vasc Surg. 2008;48:918-25, discussion 925.
20. Higuera F, Rosenthal VD, Duarte P, Ruiz J, Franco G, Safdar N. The effect of process control on the incidence of central venous catheter-associated bloodstream infections and mortality in intensive care units in Mexico. Crit Care Med. 2005;33:2022-7.
21. Karakitsos D, et al. Real-time ultrasound-guided catheterisation of the internal jugular vein: a prospective comparison with the landmark technique in critical care patients. Crit Care. 2006;10:R162.
22. Lorente L, Henry C, Martín MM, Jime´nez A, Mora ML. Central venous catheter-related infection in a prospective and observational study of 2,595 catheters. Crit Care. 2005;9:R631-5.
23. Marino PL. Establishing venous access. In: Marino PL, Sutin KM, editors. The ICU book. 3rd Edition. Philadelphia: Lippincott, Williams & Wilkins; 2007.p.107-28.
24. McKinley S, Mackenzie A, Finfer S, Ward R, Penfold J. Incidence and predictors of central venous catheter related infection in intensive care patients. Anaesth Intensive Care. 1999;27:164-9.
25. Merrer J, De Jonghe B, Golliot F, Lefrant JY, Raffy B, Barre E, et atl. French Catheter Study Group in Intensive Care: Complications of femoral and subclavian venous catheterization in critically ill patients: A randomized controlled trial. JAMA 2001;286:700-7.
26. Miller AH, Roth BA, Mills TJ, et al. Ultrasound guidance versus the landmark technique for the placement of central venous catheters in the emergency department. Acad Emerg Med. 2002;9:800.
27. Miller MR, Griswold M, Harris JM 2nd, Yenokyan G, Huskins WC, Moss M, et al. Decreasing PICU catheter-associated bloodstream infections: NACHRI's quality transformation efforts. Pediatrics. 2010;125:206-13.

28. Modeliar SS, Sevestre MA, de Cagny B, Slama M. Ultrasound evaluation of central veins in the intensive care unit: Effects of dynamic manoeuvres. Intensive Care Med. 2008;34:333-8.
29. Molgaard O, Nielsen MS, Handberg BB, Jensen JM, Kjaergaard J, Juul N. Routine X-ray control of upper central venous lines: Is it necessary? Acta Anaesthesiol Scand. 2004;48:685-9.
30. Moore C. Ultrasound-guided procedures in emergency medicine. Ultrasound Clin. 2011;6:277-89.
31. Nevarre DR, Domingo OH. Supraclavicular approach to subclavian catheterization: review of the literature and results of 178 attempts by the same operator. J Trauma. 1997;42(2):305-9.
32. Parienti JJ, du Cheyron D, Ramakers M, Malbruny B, Leclercq R, Le Coutour X, et al. Members of the NACRE Study Group: Alcoholic providone-iodine to prevent central venous catheter colonization: A randomized unit crossover study. Crit Care Med. 2004;32:708-13.
33. Parienti JJ, Thirion M, et al. Members of the Cathedia Anesthesiology 2012; Femoral vs jugular venous catheterization and risk of nosocomial events in adults requiring acute renal replacement therapy: A randomized controlled trial. JAMA. 2008;299:2413-22.
34. Parry G. Trendelenburg position, head elevation and a midline position optimize right internal jugular vein diameter. Can J Anaesth. 2004;51:379-81.
35. Pronovost P, Needham D, Berenholtz S, Sinopoli D, Chu H, Cosgrove S, et al. An intervention to decrease catheterrelated bloodstream infections in the ICU. N Engl J Med. 2006;355:2725-32.
36. Rupp SM, Apfelbaum JL, Blitt C, Caplan RA, Connis RT, Domino KB, et al. Practice guidelines for central venous access: A report by the American Society of Anaesthesiologists Task Force on Central Venous Access: Anaesthesioly. 2012;116;539-73.
37. Schnadower D, Lin S, Perera P, Smerling A, Dayan P. A pilot study of ultrasound analysis before pediatric

peripheral vein cannulation attempt. Acad Emerg Med. 2007;14:483-5.
38. Schulman J, Stricof R, Stevens TP, Horgan M, Gase K, Holzman IR, et al. New York State Regional Perinatal Care Centers: Statewide NICU central-line-associated bloodstream infection rates decline after bundles and checklists. Pediatrics. 2011;127:436-44.
39. Shah PM, Babu SC, Goyal A, Mateo RB, Madden RE. Arterial misplacement of large-caliber cannulas during jugular vein catheterization: Case for surgical management. Am Coll Surg. 2004;198:939-44.
40. Sierzenski PR, Gukhool J, Leech SJ. Emergency ultrasound. In: Knoop KJ, editor. The Atlas of Emergency Medicine. 3rd edition. New York: McGraw-Hill; 2010.
41. Spafford PS, Sinkin RA, Cox C, Reubens L, Powell KR. Prevention of central venous catheter-related coagulase negative staphylococcal sepsis in neonates. J Pediatr. 1994;125:259-63.
42. Suarez T, Baerwald JP, Kraus C. Central venous access: The effects of approach, position, and head rotation on internal jugular vein cross-sectional area. Anesth Analg. 2002;95:1519-24.
43. Sznajder JI, Zveibil FR, Bitterman H, Weiner P, Bursztein S. Central vein catheterization: Failure and complication rates by three percutaneous approaches. Arch Intern Med. 1986;146:259-61.
44. Tugrul M, Camci E, Pembeci K, Al-Darsani A, Telci L. Relation-Anesthesiology 2012;116:539-73 571 Practice Guidelines ship between peripheral and central venous pressures in different patient positions, catheter sizes, and insertion sitesJ Cardiothorac Vasc Anesthesia. 2004; 18:446-50.
45. Ultrasound guidance for placement of central venous catheters: Tom Ashar Israeli Journal of Emergency Medicine. 2007;7(2).
46. Ultrasound Guidence: For vascular access and regional Anaesthesia:Page no. 28-31 Brian A. Pollard Bsc, MD 2012.

47. Ultrasound Guidence: For vascular access and regional Anaesthesia: Page no.32 Brian A. Pollard Bsc, MD 2012.
48. Use of Ultrasound to guide Vascular Access procedures: Guidelines by American Institute of Ultrasound in Medicine. 2012.
49. Vassilomanolakis M, Plataniotis G, Koumakis G, Hajichrastou H, Skouteri H, Dova H, et al. Central venous catheter-related infections after bone marrow transplantation in patients with malignancies: A prospective study of short-course vancomycin prophylaxis. Bone Marrow Transplant. 1995;15:77-80.
50. Wang R, Snoey ER, Clements RC, Hern HG, Price D. Effect of head rotation on vascular anatomy of the neck: an ultrasound study. J Emerg Med 2006; 31:283-6.
51. Warren DK, Cosgrove SE, Diekema DJ, Zuccotti G, Climo MW, Bolon MK, et al. Prevension Epicenter Program: A multicenter intervention to prevent catheter-associated bloodstream infections. Infect Control Hosp Epidemiol. 2006;27:662-9.
52. Wyatt CR. Venous and intraosseus access in adults. In: Tintinalli JE, editor. Tintinalli's emergency medicine: a comprehensive study guide. New York: McGraw-Hill; 2011.
53. Yoffa D. Supraclavicular subclavian venipuncture and catheterization. Lancet. 1965;2:614-7.

Chapter 3

Complications and their Management

COMPLICATIONS OF CENTRAL VENOUS ACCESS

The complications associated with central venous access can be divided as follows:
- *Infectious*
  - Sepsis, cellulitis
- *Vascular*
  - Air embolus
  - Arterial puncture
  - Arteriovenous fistula
  - Hematoma
  - Blood clot
- *Miscellaneous*
  - Dysrhythmias
  - Catheter knotting or malposition
  - Nerve injury
  - Pneumothorax, hemothorax, hydrothorax, hemomediastinum
  - Bowel or bladder perforation.

Following are the factors determining rate of complications:
- *Experience with catheterization:* The experience of the physician is the most important factor in determining the risk of complications. Again if

catheter insertion fails after two or three attempts the physician should seek help rather than continue to attempt the procedure. There are increased chances of mechanical complications after three or more insertion attempts.
- *Ultrasound guidance:* The use of ultrasound definitely reduces the chances of complications. So in hospitals where ultrasound machine is easily available and physicians are well trained in using it, the procedure should be done under ultrasound guidance.
- *Insertion sites:* The most common site to perform procedure depends on physician's experience, but there are certain conditions where site should be chosen according to patient's condition. In morbidly obese patients in whom the landmarks of neck are often obscured. Internal jugular catheterization can be difficult, while in patients with severe hypoxemia Subclavian venous catheterization should be avoided as chances of pneumothorax are more likely to occur at this site. In patients with grossly contaminated inguinal region, femoral catheterization should be avoided to prevent infection, while it is preferred site during resuscitation from shock because of the ease with which it can be performed. In such situation internal jugular or subclavian venous catheterization will be difficult, but after resuscitation, the catheter should be replaced at the most appropriate site.

INFECTIOUS COMPLICATIONS OF CENTRAL VENOUS CATHETERIZATION AND THEIR PREVENTION

Rate of infection due to central venous access depends on insertion technique, use of prophylactic antibiotic or on type of catheter used.

Insertion Technique

While performing the procedure, one should use maximal sterile-barrier precautions, including a mask, a cap, a sterile gown, sterile gloves, and a large sterile drape. The use of chlorhexidine-based solutions for skin preparation is preferred to the use of povidone-iodine solutions, because chlorhexidine reduces the risk of catheter colonization.

The rate of infection is low at subclavian venous site compared to femoral venous catheterization and internal jugular catheterization. Thus, subclavian cannulation reduces the risk of infectious complications.

Prophylactic Antibiotics

The role of Prophylactic Antibiotics should only be considered in immunocompromised patients or neonates. Routine use of antibiotics is not recommended as it can encourage the emergence of antibiotic-resistant organisms.

Types of Catheters

Antimicrobial-Impregnated Catheters

Different types of antimicrobial-impregnated catheters are available in which catheters impregnated with chlorhexidine and silver sulfadiazine and catheters impregnated with minocycline and rifampin are the most frequently used types of catheters. These catheters can definitely reduce the rate of catheter-related bloodstream infections.

These catheters are particularly useful when the institutional rate of catheter-related bloodstream infections is higher.

Single-Lumen and Multilumen Catheters

There is no correlation between infection and number of lumina.

Maintenance of the Insertion Site

The use of antiseptic-containing hub should be used to decrease the risk of catheter-related bloodstream infections especially during prolonged catheterization.

Catheter Maintenance

When catheter is kept for more than 7 days chances of infection increases, so it is advisable to remove the catheter as soon as it is no longer needed, or if patient requires catheter over 7 days it should be either replaced using exchange over a guidewire or routine replacement at a new site should be considered.

Management of Suspected Catheter-related Bloodstream Infection

Whenever you suspect that infection is due to catheter two samples of blood from central line and peripheral line should be taken. In such conditions negative culture from a catheter rules out the presence of a catheter-related bloodstream infection. At the same time look at the catheter site for purulence or erythema.

If any signs of either sepsis or septic shock are found then empirical antibiotic therapy for *Staphylococcus epidermidis* or *S. aureus* infections should be started.

For immunocompromised patient antibiotic therapy for Gram-negative organisms should be added.

MECHANICAL COMPLICATIONS

- Arterial puncture, hematoma, and pneumothorax are the most common mechanical complications

during the catheterization of internal jugular vein and subclavian vein. Overall, internal jugular catheterization and subclavian venous catheterization carry similar risks of mechanical complications. Subclavian catheterization is more likely than internal jugular catheterization to be complicated by pneumothorax and hemothorax, whereas internal jugular catheterization is more likely to be associated with arterial puncture.
- Hematoma and arterial puncture are common during femoral venous catheterization.

Complications	Internal jugular vein	Subclavian vein	Femoral vein
Infection	Less chances	Less chances	Highest risk of infection
Arterial puncture and hematoma	Can occur, here bleeding can be recognized easily and can be compressed	Can occur here bleeding cannot be recognized easily and difficult to compress the vessel as it lies beneath the clavicle	Can occur
Pneumothorax	With high approach less chances with lower approach pneumothorax can occur	Highest risk of pneumothorax should be avoided in intubated patients and children less than 2 years	No risk of pneumothorax
DVT	No risk	No risk	Risk of DVT
Catheter malposition	Rare	Rare	Not good for ambulatory patients

Abbreviation: DVT, deepvein thrombosis

Recognition of Arterial Puncture

Arterial puncture in normotensive patient can be identified by pulsatile flow and bright red color of blood but in patients with profound hypotension and desaturation it becomes difficult to recognize arterial flow. In a patient with normal blood pressure and normal arterial oxygen tension, arterial puncture is usually easy to identify by the pulsatile flow into the syringe and the bright-red color of the blood.

However, in patients with profound hypotension or marked arterial desaturation, these findings may not be present. In such conditions catheter should be inserted over the wire and then can be connected to a pressure transducer to look for the venous waveforms and venous pressure, at the same time collect the blood samples for blood gas analysis. This will help to differentiate artery from vein. Again ultrasound is very much useful in this condition.

Prevention of Air Embolism

While cannulating internal jugular vein or subclavian vein patient should be placed in Trendelenburg position, and catheter hubs should be occluded at all times to prevent air embolism.

If patient develops air embolism then place the patient in Trendelenburg's position with a left lateral decubitus tilt to prevent the movement of air into the right ventricle. If the tip of catheter is located in the right atrium, aspirate the air.

MANAGEMENT OF ARTERIAL TRAUMA OR INJURY DUE TO CENTRAL VENOUS CATHETERIZATION

- When accidental cannulation of an arterial vessel occurs, the dilator or catheter should be left in place

and a general surgeon, a vascular surgeon, or an interventional radiologist should be immediately consulted regarding surgical or nonsurgical catheter removal for adults
- Once the injury has been evaluated and a treatment plan has been executed, the anesthesiologist and surgeon should consider relative risks and benefits of proceeding with the elective surgery versus deferring surgery to allow for a period of patient observation.

THROMBOTIC COMPLICATIONS

Thrombotic complications are high with femoral vein than internal jugular vein and found least with subclavian vein.

BIBLIOGRAPHY

1. Bock SN, Lee RE, Fisher B, et al. A prospective randomized trial evaluating prophylactic antibiotics to prevent triple-lumen catheter-related sepsis in patients treated with immunotherapy. J Clin Oncol. 1990;8:161-9.
2. Bold RJ, Winchester DJ, Madary AR, Gregurich MA, Mansfield PF. Prospective, randomized trial of Doppler-assisted subclavian vein catheterization. Arch Surg. 1998;133:1089-93.
3. Clark-Christoff N, Watters VA, Sparks W, Snyder P, Grant JP. Use of triple-lumen subclavian catheters for administration of total parenteral nutrition. J Parenter Enteral Nutr. 1992;16:403-7.
4. Fares LG II, Block PH, Feldman SD. Improved house staff results with subclavian cannulation. Am Surg. 1986;52:108-11.
5. Heard SO, Wagle M, Vijayakumar E, et al. Influence of triple-lumen central venous catheters coated with chlorhexidine and silver sulfadiazine on the incidence of catheter-related bacteremia. Arch Intern Med. 1998;158:81-7.

6. Hirsch DR, Ingenito EP, Goldhaber SZ. Prevalence of deep venous thrombosis among patients in medical intensive care. JAMA. 1995;274:335-7.
7. Lefrant JY, Cuvillon P, Benezet JF, et al. Pulsed Doppler ultrasonography guidance for catheterization of the subclavian vein: a randomized study. Anesthesiology. 1998;88:1195-201.
8. Maki DG, Stolz SM, Wheeler S, Mermel LA. Prevention of central venous catheter-related bloodstream infection by use of an antiseptic-impregnated catheter: a randomized, controlled trial. Ann Intern Med. 1997;127:257-66.
9. Ma TY, Yoshinaka R, Banaag A, Johnson B, Davis S, Berman SM. Total parenteral nutrition via multilumen catheters does not increase the risk of catheter-related sepsis: a randomized, prospective study. Clin Infect Dis. 1998;27:500-3.
10. McGee DC, Gould MK. Preventing Complications of Central Venous Catheterization. N Engl J Med. 2003;348:1123-33. DOI: March 20 : 200310.1056/NEJMra011883.
11. McKinley S, Mackenzie A, Finfer S, Ward R, Penfold J. Incidence and predictors of central venous catheter related infection in intensive care patients. Anaesth Intensive Care. 1999;27:164-9.
12. Raad I, Darouiche R, Dupuis J, et al. Central venous catheters coated with minocycline and rifampin for the prevention of catheter-related colonization and bloodstream infections: a randomized, double-blind trial. Ann Intern Med. 1997;127:267-74.
13. Raad I, Darouiche R, Dupuis J, et al. Central venous catheters coated with minocycline and rifampin for the prevention of catheter-related colonization and bloodstream infections: a randomized, double-blind trial. Ann Intern Med. 1997;127:267-74.
14. Randolph AG, Cook DJ, Gonzales CA, Pribble CG. Ultrasound guidance for placement of central venous catheters: a meta-analysis of the literature. Crit Care Med. 1996;24:2053-8.

15. Recommendations for preventing the spread of vancomycin resistance: recommendations of the Hospital Infection Control Practices Advisory Committee (HICPAC). MMWR Morb Mortal Wkly Rep. 1995;44:1-13.
16. Rupp SM, Connis RT, et al. Practise guidelines for central venous access: A report by the American Society of Anaesthesiologists Task Force on Central Venous Access. Anaesthesiolgoy. 2012;116:539-73.
17. Sznajder JI, Zveibil FR, Bitterman H, Weiner P, Bursztein S. Central vein catheterization: failure and complication rates by three percutaneous approaches. Arch Intern Med. 1986;146:259-61.
18. Teichgraber UK, Benter T, Gebel M, Manns MP. A sonographically guided technique for central venous access. Am J Roentgenol. 1997;169:731-3.
19. Timsit JF, Farkas JC, Boyer JM, et al. Central vein catheter-related thrombosis in intensive care patients: incidence, risk factors, and relationship with catheter-related sepsis. Chest. 1998;114:207-13.
20. Venus B, Satish P. Vascular cannulation. In: Civetta JM, Taylor RW, Kirby RR, (Eds). Critical Care. (3rd edn). Philadelphia: Lippincott-Raven, 1997:521-44.

Chapter 4

Ultrasound-guided Peripheral Venous Access

PERIPHERAL VENOUS ACCESS

Introduction
- Peripheral veins are usually easy to access directly but in certain conditions like burns, trauma, obesity it may be difficult to access directly peripheral vein, in such conditions deep veins which are not visualized or felt can be cannulated using ultrasound
- Usually peripheral veins are easily seen but sometimes if it lying deep they can be made prominent by dependent position or by applying tourniquet proximally. They are thin walled.

Important Points to Cannulate Peripheral Veins
- Peripheral veins are easily accessed at "branch points" where two smaller veins merge into a larger one
- Always start with distal veins before proximal ones
- The upper extremity is preferred to the lower extremity
- Do not attempt over a joint—for catheter security, to improve flow through the catheter, and for maximum patient comfort and mobility

- Avoid peripheral venous access through overlying infected skin, or in the same extremity as a significant traumatic injury, burn, or edema
- Avoid cannulation of an extremity with an arteriovenous fistula or other dialysis access.

Indications and Contraindications

- For medication or intravenous contrast administration
- Laboratory testing of venous blood, fluid resuscitation in situations like shock, trauma.

Peripheral cannulation should be avoided when sclerosing or vasoactive medications or extraordinarily concentrated solutions need to be infused. In such conditions central venous access is preferred.

Special Considerations, Complications, and Pearls and Pitfalls

- External jugular vein or deep brachial vein is preferred first when other sites for peripheral veins are difficult
- While performing procedure under ultrasound guidance veins are seen as black (fluid-filled, hypoechoic) circular structures that are nonpulsatile and easily compressible.

Following are certain conditions where ultrasound will be very much helpful for peripheral venous line placement.
- Obesity
- Dark-skinned patient
- An intravenous drug abuser
- At the extremes of age
- Hypotensive patient
- Patient having multiple injuries limiting the number of limbs available for use
- Patients on chemotherapy

- Patients with end-stage renal disease
- Nursing home patients with multiple IV scars
- The upper limb peripheral cannulation is the preferred site over lower limb because of the increased incidence of thrombophlebitis and thrombosis with lower limb infusions, as well as the need to often immobilize the patient if a drip is sited in the lower limb. The non-dominant upper limb is preferred as an initial option.

TECHNIQUE FOR ULTRASOUND-GUIDED PERIPHERAL VENOUS ACCESS

- As such technique remains same as the central venous access
- Three main peripheral veins of the antecubital region are: (1) Basilic, (2) cephalic, and (3) brachial veins (Fig. 1). Any other peripheral vein can also be cannulated under ultrasound guidance using same method
- These veins are variable in location and are surrounded by nerves. Hence, ultrasound guidance is helpful when cannulating these veins. The basilic vein passes upward and anteromedially to the elbow, where it receives the medial cubital vein. Then it continues on the medial to the biceps brachii, deep to the fascia, until it joins the brachial vein and becomes the axillary vein at the border of the teres major.

Figure 2 shows probe position for brachial vein cannulation and Figure 3 demonstrates correct positioning of the transducer for cephalic vein cannulation. The cephalic vein lies laterally in the superficial fascia of the antecubital fossa and it ascends along the lateral side of the forearm and upper arm. As with central venous access, place the transducer in the short-axis view and scan the vessels in the antecubital fossa. Move the probe from lateral to medial to assess vessel location.

Ultrasound-guided Peripheral Venous Access

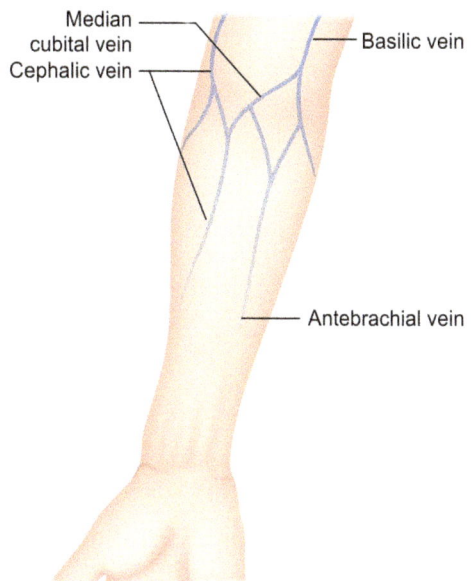

Fig. 1: Anatomic positioning of the major vessels of the antecubital region. The basilic, cephalic and brachial veins

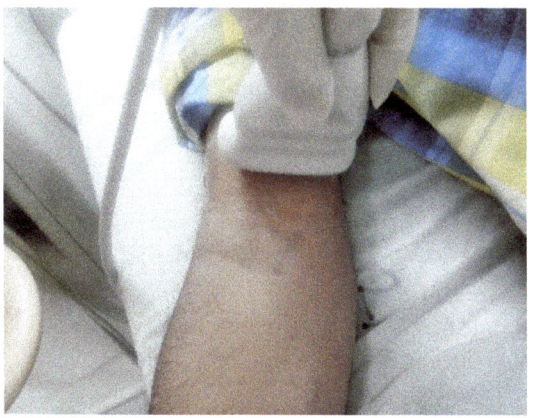

Fig. 2: Transducer position for brachial vein cannulation

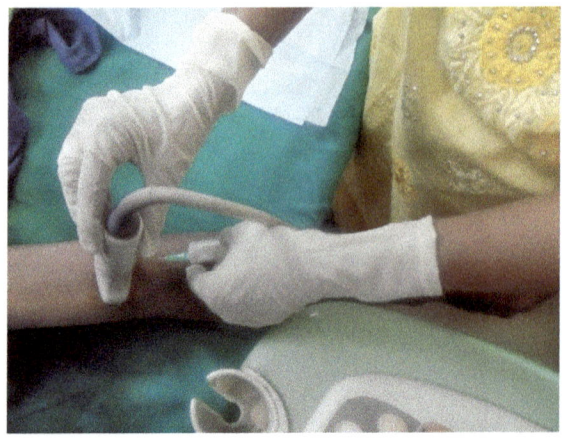

Fig. 3: Probe position for cephalic vein cannulation

Equipment Required for US-guided Peripheral Venous Access

- High-frequency linear transducer, gel
- Gloves
- Topical local anesthetic (especially for pediatric patients)
- Catheter and needle device
- Gauze, tape, and transparent dressing
- Antiseptic solution or wipe
- Tourniquet
- IV tubing, flushes, syringe.

Technique for Peripheral Venous Access

- *Position of the patient:* Patient should be positioned in supine position with the extremity of choice extended on a flat surface, palm up
- *Transducer position:* Horizontally in antecubital fossa

- Start scanning from lateral to medial side without giving much pressure as veins are easily compressible. You may need to tilt transducer to find out the vein
- Now bring the image of vein in the middle of the screen and confirm with color Doppler
- Then insert the needle out of plane at a 45° angle to the skin
- As soon as the needle is inserted in the skin, attempt to find out the tip by sweeping distally with the probe. Aspirate to confirm the needle position
- Now thread the catheter over the needle tip to cannulate the vein and secure the catheter
- The position of catheter can also be confirmed by changing the plane of transducer.

Ultrasound Guidance for Peripherally Inserted Central Catheter

- Peripherally inserted central venous catheters (PICCs) are nowadays used as alternative to central venous access in patients requiring long-term intravenous therapy
- Advantages of the PICC include:
  - Chances of complications like air embolism, pneumothorax, DVT, major arterial puncture hence hematoma etc. are decreased compared to central venous access
  - Procedure is easy and can be performed bedside
  - Cost-effective.

Advantages of Ultrasound Guidance for PICC Placement

- Increased success rate
- Easy to visualize vessel
- Reducing the risk of arterial puncture.

Technique for Ultrasound-guided Peripherally Inserted Central Catheter Placement

- The most common site for venous access for a PICC is obtained through an antecubital vein. The success rate with basilica vein is high compared to cephalic vein as the course of cephalic vein is tortuous
- The procedure should be carried out under full antiseptic precaution same as mentioned above for basilica or cephalic vein cannulation
- The ultrasound guidance should be used to confirm the position of guidewire and catheter.

Sometimes catheter tip may move cephalic so to confirm proper position three different techniques are used:

- Ultrasound guidance helps to confirm PICC placement by visualizing agitated saline from an intravenous flush in the right atrium of the heart after placement
- Electrocardiographic guidance helps to confirm the tip position
- Post-procedure X-ray chest should be carried out.

Ultrasound Guidance for Arterial Access Procedures

Arterial access is used for invasive blood pressure monitoring as well as for procedural purposes. Ultrasound guidance helps in identifying and accessing the arterial lumen in patients that have good external anatomic landmarks as well as in patients whose external landmarks are less well-defined.

US-guidance for arterial access is particularly useful:
- In patients with obesity
- Altered anatomy

- Low systemic perfusion, or nonpulsatile blood flow
- Patients in whom previous cannulation attempts have been unsuccessful.

Common sites for arterial access include femoral, radial, brachial, axillary, and dorsalis pedis arteries.

The radial artery cannulation is safe because of its accessibility, predictable location, and low complication rates associated with both its access and use. It is usually easily palpable and is also not typically the sole blood supply to the distal extremity, unlike the axillary, brachial, and femoral arteries.

Technique for Ultrasound-guided Arterial Access

The technique for ultrasound-guided aterial access remains same except following points:
- Arteries should be identified and differentiated from veins using color Doppler and pulse wave Doppler
- Identification of plaque, arterial spasm, hematoma, or decreased luminal diameter with ultrasound helps to avoid futile cannulation attempts and directs the operator to a more desirable location
- For radial artery cannulation, an Allen test for collateral perfusion should be performed
- For optimal positioning of the wrist put support below the wrist joint that should include a support that allows the wrist to be approximately 45° extended (more than 45° may cause the vessel to be compressed)
- Conditions such as hypotension, low cardiac output, and an excessive limb circumference that contribute to arterial cannulation failures with a landmark-guided technique may be equally challenging despite ultrasound guidance
- The rest of the procedure is same as in central and peripheral venous cannulation.

BIBLIOGRAPHY

1. Feldman R. General principles of intravenous access. In: Reichman EF, Simon RR (Eds). Emergency medicine procedures. New York: McGraw-Hill; 2004;314-37.
2. Keyes LE, Frazee BW, Snoey ER, et al. Ultrasound-guided brachial and basilica vein cannulation in emergency department patients with difficult intravenous access. Ann Emerg Med. 1999;34(6):711.
3. Lewis GC, et al. Critical skills and Procedures in Emergency Medicine: Vascular Access skills and procedures. Emerg Med Clin North Am. 2013;31(1):59-86.
4. Mbamalu D, Banerjee A. Methods of obtaining peripheral venous access in difficult situations. Postgrad Med. 1999;75(886):459.
5. Reichman EF, Oakes JL. Vascular access. In: Wolfson AB, (Ed). Harwood-Nuss' Clinical Practice of Emergency Medicine. 4th edition. Philadelphia: Lippincott Williams & Wilkins; 2005;43-55.
6. Roseman JM. Deep, percutaneous antecubital venipuncture: an alternative to surgical cutdown. Am J Surg. 1983;146(2):285.
7. Sierzenski PR, Gukhool J, Leech SJ. Emergency ultrasound. In: Knoop KJ, (Ed). The Atlas of Emergency Medicine. 3rd edition. New York: McGraw-Hill; 2010.
8. Stroud S, Rodriguez R. Arterial puncture and cannulation. In: Reichman EF, Simon RR, (Eds). Emergency Medicine Procedures. New York: McGraw-Hill; 2004;398-410.

Chapter 5

Introduction of Ultrasound-guided Regional Block

HISTORY

Modern local analgesia began with the introduction of cocaine into medical practice in 1884 by Kollar. Within 1 year, William Halsted and Richard Hall introduced cocaine by performing the first successful nerve block of the infraorbital plexus. The major drawbacks of cocaine were its toxicity and addiction, so, alternative agents were invented.

Procaine (Novocain®) was discovered by Alfred Einhorn in 1904 and became the local anesthetic of choice for 40 years. The disadvantages of procaine, short duration of action and high rate of allergic reactions, prompted the search for an alternative local anesthetic agent. Lidocaine was introduced by Nils Löfgren in 1943 and continues to be the local anesthetic of choice today.

The term Regional Anesthesia was first used by Harvey Cushing (1869-1939) in 1901 to describe pain relief by nerve block.

Nowadays Anesthesiologists routinely perform peripheral nerve blocks for a wide variety of procedures. The basic principle of a peripheral nerve block is to apply a local anesthetic directly on to a peripheral nerve or nerve plexus to completely anesthetize the surgical site.

To start with anesthesiologists have performed peripheral nerve blocks using the anatomical landmark technique (paresthesia technique), in which the needle is inserted at a point determined by standard anatomic landmarks and then advanced until the patient feels paresthesia in the relevant sensory distribution. Later on in the 1970s and 1980s, anesthesiologists started using a peripheral nerve stimulator to locate nerve. Since past two decades, ultrasound has gained much popularity to improve nerve localization.

The advantages of ultrasound over other two techniques are as follows:
- Using ultrasound we can directly visualize the nerve of interest, the needle tip itself and the spread of the local anesthetic drug around the plexus
- Ultrasound also helps to visualize other surrounding structures such as blood vessels and lungs, so that we can avoid the complications like intravascular injection or pneumothorax
- At last it improves the overall success rate of the procedures, their safety and speed.

LOCAL ANESTHETIC AGENTS

Local anesthetic agents are the *medication* that causes reversible loss of *pain* sensation, although other senses like loss of muscle power are often affected as well. Clinical local anesthetics belong to one of two classes: aminoamide and aminoester local anesthetics. Synthetic local anesthetics are structurally related to *cocaine*. They differ from cocaine mainly in that they have a very low abuse potential and do not produce *hypertension* or (with few exceptions) *vasoconstriction*.

Local Anesthetic Agents

Agent	Duration (min)	Onset (min)	Maximum dose mg/kg (with epinephrine)	Concentration
Amides				
Bupivacaine	200+	10–15	3	0.25–0.50%
Lidocaine	30–60	5	4(7)	1–2%, (5% for spinal anesthesia)
Levobupivacaine	200+	10–15	2	0.50%
Mepivacaine	45–90	3	4	1–2%
Prilocaine	30–90	5	5	4%
Ropivacaine	200+	5–15	3	0.5%
Esters				
Procaine	40	15–20	7	0.5–2.0%
Chlorprocaine	45	5	8	1–2%
Tetracaine	200	15	1.5	0.2–0.3%

Techniques

Different methods used for local anesthesia are as follows:

- *Spinal and epidural anesthesia:* These are central neuraxial blocks, that anesthesiologist routinely uses
- *Surface anesthesia:* Local anesthetic is used as spray, solution or cream over the skin or a mucous membrane. The effect lasts for a short duration
- *Infiltration anesthesia:* Here the local anesthetic is infiltraed into the tissue to be anesthetized
- *Field block:* In this technique local anesthetic is injected subcutaneously in the border of area to be anesthetized

- *Peripheral nerve block:* In this technique local anesthetic is injected in the vicinity of a peripheral nerve to block the area supplied by that nerve
- *Plexus anesthesia:* Here local anesthetic is injected in the vicinity of a nerve plexus. It blocks whole area innervated by that plexus
- Other techniques are Intravenous regional anesthesia (Bier's block), Intrapleural anesthesia, Intraarticular anesthesia, etc.

REGIONAL ANESTHESIA

Regional anesthesia is a technique that infiltrates local anesthetic agents adjacent to peripheral nerves (nerve blocks).

Regional anesthesia is mainly used for complicated lacerations, fractures, and dislocations.

Preparation for Regional Blocks

- Always insert an intravenous line before commencing a block
- Always apply monitor—pulse oximetry, EGG, BP—as indicated
- Always practice proper aseptic technique
- Always have resuscitation equipment at hand
- Always obtain the patients informed consent
- Always have an adequate knowledge of the correct technique
- Know how to handle complications.

Advantages of Regional Anesthesia

- The complications related to general anesthesia like trauma to lips, teeth, oropharynx and vocal cords, bronchospasm, aspiration, prolonged sedation can be avoided

Introduction of Ultrasound-guided Regional Block

- It is safer than general anesthesia particularly in inexperienced hands and remote locations
- Patient remains awake during surgery so can interact with the surgeon
- There are less chances of sedation, nausea and vomiting postoperatively
- Intraoperatively there is decreased stress response to surgery and blood loss
- There are decreased chances of deep vein thrombosis with spinal anesthesia.

Disadvantages of Regional Anesthesia

- Procedure for regional anesthesia and its onset takes time around 15–30 minutes
- Patient may feel discomfort due to procedure and positioning
- Some patients may remain anxious and dislike being aware
- Some surgeons get distracted by awake patient
- Anesthetist should have proper knowledge, skill and equipment before performing the procedure
- There are chances of block failure and permanent nerve damage.

Complications of Regional Anesthesia

Complications of regional anesthesia are not serious but sometimes it can be life-threatening.

Local Anesthesia Toxicity

When the concentration of local anesthetic in the blood rises to a toxic level local anesthetic toxicity can occur.

Signs and Symptoms

- Early symptoms of local anesthetic toxicity include tinnitus, light headedness, facial numbness, a

metallic taste and blurred vision. Patients may become confused and disorientated. Nausea or vomiting may occur
- When serum level increases more nystagmus, tremors and isolated muscle twitching occur. This can lead to convulsions, coma and respiratory arrest
- When epinephrine is added in the local anesthetic (LA) solution, the initial signs of an overdose may be a tachycardia and hypertension. If epinephrine is not added, the early signs may be bradycardia and hypotension
- Bupivacaine is particularly dangerous as it causes a ventricular fibrillation, it can be difficult to defibrillate
- Management:
  - First secure the airway, to start with bag and mask oxygen (with high flow oxygen) but if not maintaining suxamethonium should be given followed by intubation. IPPV should be given till patient becomes conscious and is able to maintain his own airway
  - Convulsions can be managed with intravenous Benzodiazepines
  - If cardiovascular collapse occurs give intravenous atropine to reverse the bradycardia and vasodilation. Give intravenous fluids for hypotension and cardiopulmonary resuscitation if cardiac arrest occurs.
- **Prevention is always better than cure and it is advisable to adopt a few sensible practices:**
  - Inject local anesthetics slowly, aspirating every 3–5 mL
  - Stabilize the needle during injection by placing a short length of fine bore plastic tubing between the needle and syringe (the isolated needle technique)
  - Always perform a check aspiration before injecting LA (but remember, check aspirations are not foolproof)

Introduction of Ultrasound-guided Regional Block

- Observe the patient, pulse and ECG for signs of intravascular injection. Added epinephrine causes a sudden tachycardia
- Always secure intravenous access before commencing block
- Always have emergency resuscitation equipment on hand and know how to use it.

Nerve Damage

- Nerve damage can occur by direct needle trauma or by injecting local anesthetic into the nerve
- When short bevel needle is used it may contuse a nerve and when sharp needle is used it will lacerate it. When paresthesia is elicited, it is good practise to withdraw the needle a millimeter or two before injecting

Following are some tips to reduce nerve damage:
- Use short bevel needles
- Use nerve stimulators and insulated short bevel needles wherever possible
- Rapid and forceful injections should be avoided. Do not inject against high resistance
- When the patient is under anesthesia avoid regional anesthesia.

Infection

- Always use strict aseptic technique. This means sterile gloves, drapes and an appropriate prep solution
- Do not introduce needle through infected skin.

Hematoma

If patient has any coagulopathy or bleeding disorder, be careful while giving subarachnoid block, Extradural block or plexus block.

Methods for Regional Blocks

Regional blocks can be given using different techniques.
- Using anatomical landmark technique
- Using peripheral nerve locator
- Regional block under ultrasound guidance.

Table shows advantages and disadvantages of each technique.

TABLE 1: Advantages and disadvantages of different techniques

Method	Advantages	Disadvantages
Landmark technique	Cost effective	Anatomic variation. Large volumes of anesthetic are typically administered
Peripheral nerve locator technique	Reduces the number of needle passes	If high frequency chosen will produce pain in the muscles
US-guided technique	1. Shortens the block performance time 2. Reduces the no. of needle passes 3. Enables blocks to be performed using low anesthetic doses	1. Equipments are costly 2. Expertise is required 3. Hand-eye coordination is required

Routine Monitors

- Pulse oximetry
- Noninvasive blood pressure
- Electrocardiogram
- Respiratory rate
- Mental status (BIS monitor).

Emergency drugs required during nerve block procedures:
- Atropine
- Ephedrine
- Phenylephrine

- Midazolam
- Propofol
- Muscle relaxant
- Thiopentone sodium.

Equipment needed includes the following:
- Ultrasound machine with linear transducer (8–14 MHz), sterile sleeve, and gel (or other coupling medium, e.g. saline)
- Standard nerve block tray
- 20 to 25 mL local anesthetic
- 5 cm, 22 gauge short-bevel insulated stimulating needle
- Peripheral nerve stimulator
- Sterile gloves.

Keep routine resuscitation kit ready.

ULTRASOUND-GUIDED REGIONAL BLOCKS

The introduction of ultrasound techniques for regional anesthesia is currently a focus for anesthesia education.

Advantages of Ultrasound

- It is portable, free of radiation risk, and relatively inexpensive when compared with other imaging modalities, such as magnetic resonance (MRI) and computed tomography (CT)
- Using ultrasound we can directly visualize the image, so that procedure can be performed under ultrasound guidance
- Using ultrasound we can also visualize the distribution of the injected medication. Thus US guidance improves the success rate of the procedures, their safety and speed
- Under ultrasound guidance we can also visualize the soft tissue

- US machine is more portable and less expensive compared to CT scan and MRI
- Thus, US-guided regional block has following benefits:
  - Optimize nerve localization
  - Visualize surrounding structures
  - Assess proper needle placement
  - Identify anomalous anatomy and pathology
  - Visualize local anesthetic spread
  - Safer compared to blind injections
  - Faster performance time
  - Fewer complications
  - Less patient discomfort
  - Enhancement of the quality of nerve blocks and longer duration.

Disadvantages of Ultrasound

- When we are doing procedure under ultrasound guidance one should have thorough knowledge of gross or micro-anatomy
- We should have gross idea of US image of a targeted structure (textbook picture), but sometimes there can be anatomic variation so that should be kept in mind
- Thus, expertise is must for performing different block.

Ultrasound-guided Upper Extremity Nerve Blocks

- Brachial plexus block:
  - Interscalene approach
  - Supraclavicular approach
  - Axillary approach
  - Infraclavicular approach
- Wrist block
- Forearm block.

Ultrasound-guided Lower Extremity Nerve Blocks

- Femoral nerve block
- Sciatic popliteal nerve block
- Ankle block.

Ultrasound-guided Other Blocks

Transverse abdominis plane block.

BIBLIOGRAPHY

1. Atkinson RS, Rushman GB, Davies NHJ. Lee's Synopsis of Anaeshesia, Eleventh edition, 1913.
2. Ihnatsenka B, Boezaart AP. Ultrasound: Basic understanding and learning the language. Int J Shoulder Surg. 2010;4(3): 55-62.

Chapter 6

Upper Extremity Nerve Blocks

Historically, anesthesiologists have performed peripheral nerve blocks using the paresthesia technique, in which the needle is inserted at a point determined by standard anatomic landmarks and then advanced until the patient feels paresthesia in the relevant sensory distribution.

In the 1970s and 1980s, anesthesiologists began using a nerve stimulator to improve needle localization.

Essentially, a nerve stimulator is a device that sends current through the block needle to elicit contraction of relevant muscle groups when in close proximity to the nerve of interest. These techniques are effective and are still in use, although they have many drawbacks.

Over the past decade, ultrasound has gained popularity for peripheral nerve blockade because it allows the anesthesiologist to directly visualize the nerves of interest, the needle tip itself, and the spread of the local anesthetic in the desired location.

In addition, the ultrasound image reliably depicts other structures such as blood vessels and lungs that the anesthesiologist wants to avoid. For these reasons, ultrasound guidance has increasingly become the standard technique for regional anesthesia.

Following are the benefits of ultrasound guided regional blocks:
- Optimization of nerve localization

- We can visualize surrounding structures
- Assess proper needle placement
- Identify anomalous anatomy and pathology
- Visualize local anesthetic spread
- Safer compared to blind injections
- Faster performance time
- Fewer complications
- Less patient discomfort
- Enhancement of the quality of nerve blocks and longer duration.

Equipment needed for ultrasound-guided regional block are as follows: Ultrasound machine with linear transducer (8–14 MHz), sterile sleeve, and gel

- Standard nerve block tray
- 5 cm, 22 gauge short-bevel insulated stimulating needle
- Peripheral nerve stimulator
- Sterile gloves.

In this chapter, we will discuss about different approaches of brachia plexus block and forearm block under ultrasound guidance.

BRACHIAL PLEXUS BLOCK

Anatomy of Brachial Plexus (Fig. 1)

The brachial plexus is formed from the anterior primary divisions of C5, C6, C7, C8 and T1. It forms the entire motor and almost the entire sensory nerve supply to arm. It receives communicating branches from C4 and T2. These nerves unite to form three trunks, which lie in the neck above the clavicle. Its roots pass through the fascia enclosed space between the scalenus anterior and scalenus medius. As the plexus converges on the first rib it is enclosed in a fibrous sheath of scalene muscles.

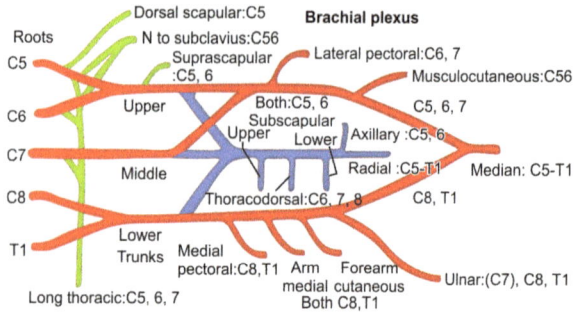

Fig. 1: Anatomy of brachial plexus

It lies first above and then to the outer sides of the subclavian vessels just above the clavicle.

The upper trunk is formed by the anterior rami of C5 and C6.

The middle trunk is formed by the anterior ramus of C7.

The lower trunk is formed by the anterior rami of C8 and T1.

Behind the clavicle the trunks each divide into anterior and posterior divisions in relation to the axillary artery.

The posterior cord is formed by the three posterior divisions.

The medial cord is formed by the lowest anterior division.

The lateral cord is formed by the upper two anterior divisions. Then branches are given off from (1) roots, (2) trunks, and (3) cords.

The brachial plexus block can be given by four different approaches (Fig. 2).
1. Interscalene approach.
2. Supraclavicular approach.
3. Axillary approach.
4. Infraclavicular approach.

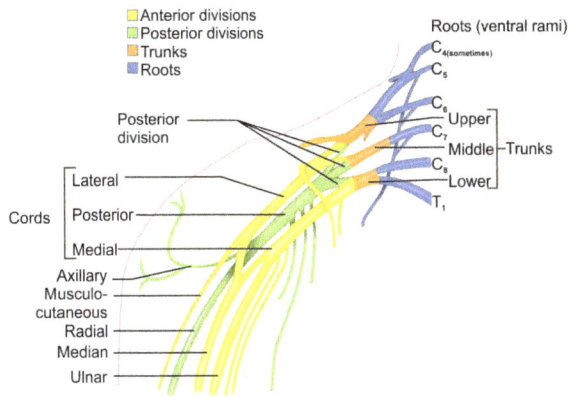

Fig. 2: Organization of the brachial plexuss

Ultrasound-guided Interscalene Brachial Plexus Block

Indications
- Interscalene block is indicated for shoulder and upper arm surgery.
- Volume of local anesthetic required: 15–25 mL.

Advantages
- Shoulder and upper arm surgery can be performed under Interscalene block.
- Dangers of pneumothorax are avoided.

Disadvantages
- There is a risk of injection into the extradural space, into CSF or vertebral artery.
- There is also risk of bilateral cervical and brachial plexus block.

Specific considerations: The most proximal approach of brachial plexus is interscalene approach. Here the roots of the plexus particularly C_3-C_7 are blocked, but sparing of the C_8 and T_1 roots occur. Thus interscalene approach of brachial plexus blocks the skin and deep structures of the shoulder, the upper arm, the elbow and the lateral aspect of the forearm and hand while structures in the medial aspect of the forearm and hand may be spared.

The ultrasound-guided technique of interscalene brachial plexus block differs from nerve stimulator or landmark-based techniques in several important aspects.

- In nerve stimulation technique usually we inject single large volume of local anesthetic at one place where chances of failure are increased but with ultrasound guidance we give multiple injections around the brachial plexus, increasing the success rate.
- Less volume is required to accomplish the block with ultrasound compared to landmark technique.
- If block fails we can also repeat the procedure with ultrasound guidance.
- Chances of major vessel and nerve puncture during nerve block are decreased.

Anatomy at interscalene level: The brachial plexus is formed by the anterior primary divisions of C5, C6, C7, C8 and T1. It forms the entire motor and the entire sensory nerve supply to the arm. It receives branches from C4 and T2. These nerves unite to form three trunks, which lie in the neck above the clavicle. Its roots pass through the fascia-enclosed space between the scalenus anterior and the scalenus medius muscle accompanied by the subclavian artery, invaginate the scalene fascia to form a neurovascular space. The interscalene block is given between the anterior and middle scalene muscles.

Ultrasound anatomy: The main structures of interest are carotid artery, prevertebral fascia, superficial cervical plexus and sternocleidomastoid muscle. Brachial plexus

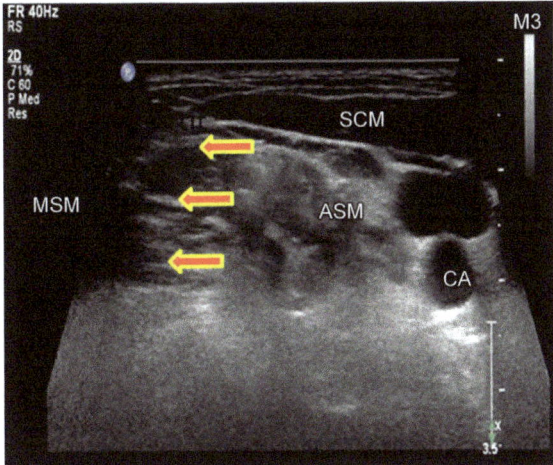

Fig. 3: Ultrasound anatomy of brachial plexus at interscalene level
Abbreviations: SCM, sternocleidomastoid muscle; ASM, anterior scalene muscle; MSM, middle scalene muscle; BP, brachial plexus; CA, carotid artery

lies between the anterior and middle scalene muscles lateral to the carotid artery. We can visualize Prevertebral fascia, superficial cervical plexus and sternocleidomastoid muscle superficial to the plexus, (Fig. 3)

Landmarks and patient positioning
- ***Patient position:*** The block should be performed in supine position, with 45° bed elevation and the patient's head turned to the opposite side.
- ***Transducer position:*** Transverse on neck, 3–4 cm superior to clavicle, over external jugular vein (Fig. 4).
- ***Technique of interscalene approach under ultrasound guidance (Fig. 5):*** After proper positioning and sterile precaution start scanning just below the level of the cricoid cartilage and medial to the sternocleidomastoid muscle to find out carotid artery.

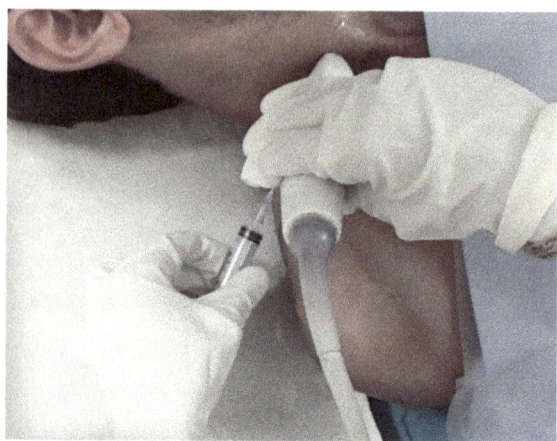

Fig. 4: Transducer position for interscalene block

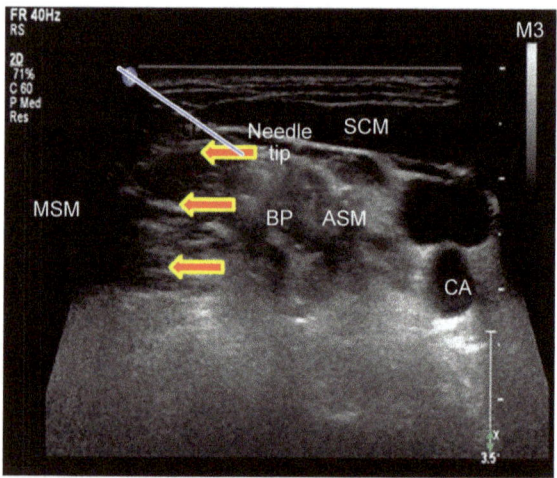

Fig. 5: Technique of interscalene approach of brachial plexus
Abbreviations: SCM, sternocleidomastoid muscle; ASM, anterior scalene; MSM, middle scalene muscle; BP, brachial plexus; CA, carotid artery

Once the artery is identified, move the transducer slightly laterally across the neck to identify the sternocleidomastoid muscle, middle and anterior scalene muscles. The brachial plexus will be seen sandwiched between the anterior and middle scalene muscles.

Insert the needle in-plane toward the brachial plexus, typically in a lateral-to-medial direction (Fig. 4). Once you insert the needle first give off of prevertebral fascia will be felt. It is difficult to visualize needle tip under ultrasound so inject 1 to 2 mL of local anesthetic to locate needle tip.

Another method is that you use nerve stimulator to confirm the needle tip position. Once confirmed the needle tip position inject rest of the local anesthetic volume that is 15 to 25 mL. While injecting drug, be careful that high resistance is not felt which suggest intrafascicular or intraneural injection.

If you find difficulty in identifying plexus bring the transducer downward up to supraclavicular fossa look for the subclavian artery and again bring transducer at cricoid cartilage level and try to find out brachial plexus.

Ultrasound-guided Supraclavicular Block

Indications
- Supraclavicular approach for brachial plexus is indicated for surgery on the arm, elbow, forearm, and hand
- Volume of local anesthetic required: 20–25 mL

Specific considerations
- The three trunks of brachial plexus run vertically across the surface of the first rib and lie in the brachial plexus sheath along with subclavian artery
- The brachial plexus in supraclavicular fossa lies close to the chest cavity and pleura, so chances of

pneumothorax and arterial puncture are very high under anatomical landmark technique, However, under ultrasound guidance we can easily visualize plexus, rib, pleura, and subclavian artery, thus minimizing the chances of complications
- As in supraclavicular approach trunks and divisions of the brachial plexus are blocked, the onset and quality of anesthesia is fast and complete.

Ultrasound anatomy
- The main structures to visualize are subclavian artery, parietal pleura and first rib. When we put the probe transversely above the clavicle first the pulsating subclavian artery will be seen, while the parietal pleura will be seen as a linear hyperechoic structure deep to it.
- The brachial plexus will be seen just lateral and superficial to the subclavian artery as bundle of round hypoechoic nodules (Fig. 6).

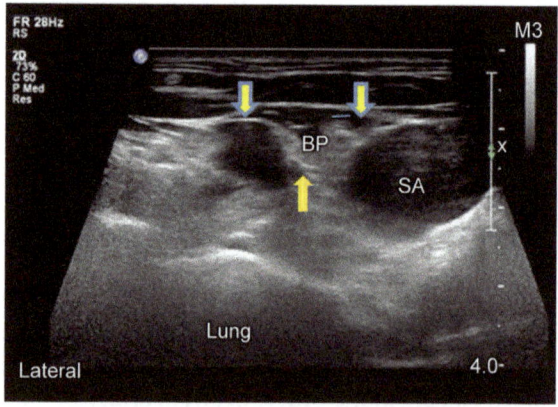

Fig. 6: Sonoanatomy of brachial plexus at supraclavicular level
Abbreviations: SA, subclavian artery; BP, brachial plexus

Upper Extremity Nerve Blocks

Landmarks and patient positioning
- ***Patient's position:*** The patient should be in supine position with head turned to the opposite side. If possible, ask the patient to stretch his hand up to the ipsilateral knee which will depress the clavicle slightly and allow better access to the structures of the anterolateral neck.
- ***Transducer position:*** Transverse on neck, just superior to the clavicle at midpoint (Fig. 7).

Technique
After giving position to the patient, and full aseptic precautions place the transducer in the transverse plane immediately superior to the clavicle at approximately its midpoint.
- Then tilt the transducer caudally to visualize first subclavian artery. Confirm the artery by using ultrasound Doppler. Immediately lateral and superficial to subclavian artery brachial plexus can be seen as bunch of grapes.
- Once identified give local anesthetic with 22- to 24-gauge needle into the skin just lateral to the

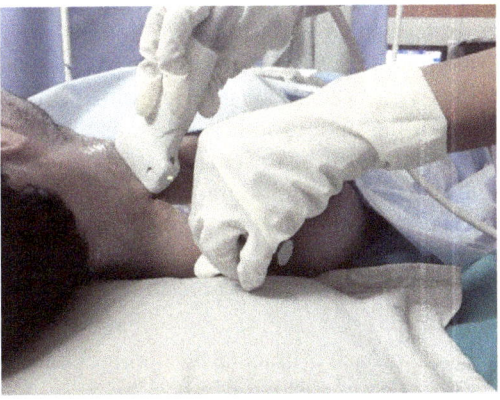

Fig. 7: Probe position for supraclavicular block

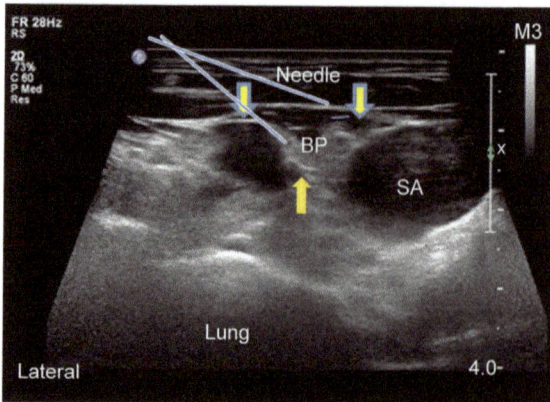

Fig. 8: Technique of supraclavicular approach of brachial plexus block
Abbreviations: BP, brachial plexus; SA, subclavian artery

transducer to decrease the discomfort to the patient.
- After that insert the needle in-plane toward the brachial plexus, in a lateral-to-medial direction. After negative aspiration, inject 1 to 2 mL of local anesthetic to confirm the needle tip.
- Always check for drug diffusion by giving small amount of local anesthetic as needle advances through tissue layers. Once confirmed placement of needle tip inject 20–25 mL local anesthetic drug at two to three different locations within plexus (Fig. 8). Do not inject the drug against resistance as it may lead to intrafascicular or intraneural injection. Confirm the spread of drug under ultrasound guidance.

Ultrasound-guided Axillary Block

Indications
- Axillary approach of brachial plexus block is indicated for surgery on forearm and hand.
- Volume of the local anesthetic required is 20–25 mL.

General considerations: This approach is safe and relatively simple method of blocking the brachial plexus, but the musculocutaneous and axillary nerve leave the sheath high in the axilla so requires additional blockade which can be done easily under ultrasound guidance.

Advantages of axillary block
- The axillary brachial plexus block is relatively simple to perform with ultrasound because of its superficial location.
- Lower risk of pneumothorax, stellate ganglion block, recurrent laryngeal nerve block or phrenic nerve block.

Anatomy: In the axilla the nerves from the brachial plexus, together with the main artery are enclosed in a fibrous neuromuscular sheath. The median and musculocutaneous nerves are anterior or anterolateral, ulnar nerve is inferior and radial nerve is posterolateral to the vessel.

Ultrasound anatomy: The main structure to visualize during axillary block is axillary artery, which lies very superficial on the anteromedial aspect of the proximal arm. Medial to artery lies axillary vein, and surrounding the artery lies all branches of brachial plexus. Lateral to the axillary artery lies median nerve, medial to the artery lies ulnar artery and radial nerve lies posterior to the artery. The fourth nerve is seen as bright hyperechoic rim as we move the transducer proximally (Fig. 9).

Technique
- **Patient position:** Patient should be in supine position with Abduction of arm at 90° (Fig. 10). Care should be taken not to overabduct the arm because that may cause discomfort as well as produce tension on the brachial plexus, making it more vulnerable to needle or injection injury during the block procedure.

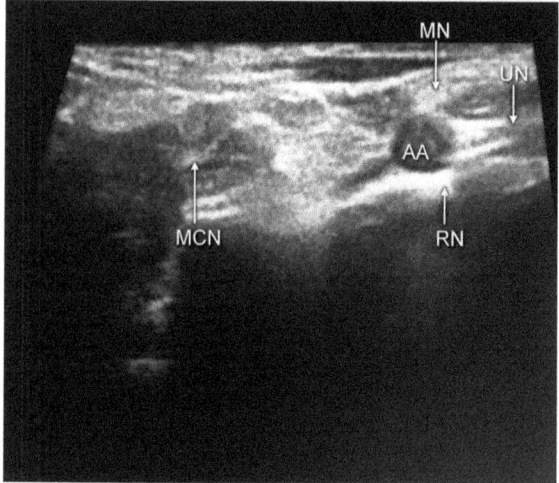

Fig. 9: Sonoanatomy of axillary approach of brachial plexus
Abbreviations: AA, axillary artery; MN, median nerve; UN, ulnar nerve; RN, radial nerve; MCN, musculocutaneous nerve

- *Transducer position:* After proper positioning of the arm Palpate the pectoralis major muscle and then place the Transducer on the skin immediately distal to that point perpendicular to the axis of the arm (Fig. 10). Initially place transducer in such a way so that it overlies both the biceps and the triceps muscles (i.e. on the medial aspect of the arm), then slide the transducer downwards across the axilla to visualize axillary artery and brachial plexus.

Technique
- After proper positioning and sterile precaution place the transducer as mentioned above. Now try to identify Axillary artery and always confirm with color Doppler and pulse wave Doppler.

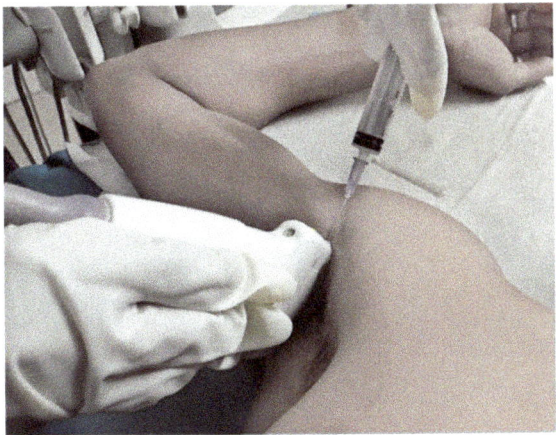

Fig. 10: Probe position for axillary block

- Now median nerve can be seen as hyperechoic rim lateral to artery, ulnar nerve can be seen medial to artery and radial nerve can be seen posterior to the artery. Insert the needle in plane first to block radial nerve posteriorly. Confirm the needle tip position by injecting 1 to 2 mL of local anesthetic and then inject 5 to 10 mL of local anesthetic injection.
- Now withdraw the needle upto skin and redirect towards ulnar and median nerve. After confirming needle tip position inject 5 to 10 mL of local anesthetic at each level.
- Then move the transducer proximally to identify musculocutaneous nerve. Again insert the needle in plane to block this nerve, inject 5 to 10 mL of local anesthetic at this level (Fig. 11). Thus total of 20 to 25 mL local anesthetic volume is required.

Important note:
- As the veins lie nearby the plexus an undue pressure with the transducer during imaging may obliterate the

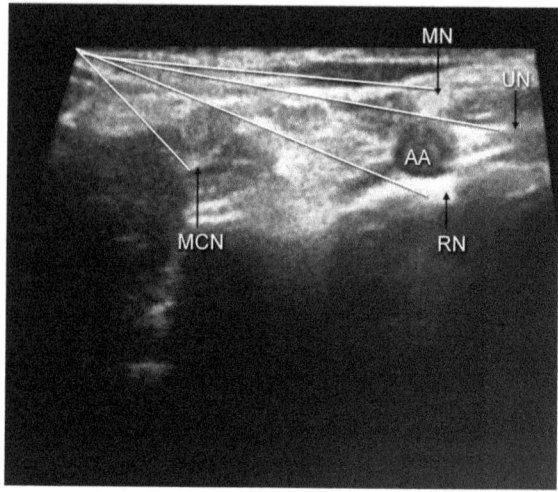

Fig. 11: Technique of axillary approach of brachial plexus block
Abbreviations: AA, axillary artery; RN, radial nerve; MN, median nerve; MCN, musculocutaneous nerve; UN, ulnar nerve

veins, rendering veins invisible and prone to puncture with the needle. So it is advisable to do frequent aspiration and slow administration of local anesthetic to decrease the risk of an intravascular injection. Keep the pressure applied on the transducer steady to avoid opening and closing of the multitude of veins in the axilla and reduce the risk of an intravascular injection.

Ultrasound-guided Infraclavicular Brachial Plexus Block

Indications
- The indications are same as axillary block, for operation on arm, elbow, forearm, and hand.
- Local anesthetic volume required is 20–30 mL.

Specific considerations: The nerve blockade with infraclavicular approach is same as axillary approach. As brachial plexus lies deep at this level long needle is required to traverse across the pectoralis major muscle, which is not comfortable to the patient and chances of pneumothorax are also high.

The only advantage of ultrasound-guided infraclavicular brachial plexus block is that identification of the arterial pulse on the sonographic image is easy, but procedure as such is difficult. The catheter placement and fixation are easier as muscles of the chest wall can stabilize catheter easily.

Ultrasound anatomy: The main structures to identify are pectoralis major muscle, pectoralis minor muscle and axillary artery. Axillary artery lies deep to the pectoralis major and minor muscles. All the three cords lateral, medial and posterior cords lie surrounding the artery. Surrounding the artery are the three cords of the brachial plexus: the lateral, posterior, and medial cords (Fig. 12).

Landmarks and patient positioning
- **Patient position:** Patient should lie in supine position with the head turned to opposite side. There should be abduction of arm at 90° and flexion of the arm which makes pectoralis muscle prominent.
- **Transducer position:** Place the transducer just below the clavicle and medial to coracoid process (Fig. 13).

Technique: After proper position and aseptic precaution place the transducer as mentioned above. The most important landmark to identify is coracoids process, which can be identified by asking the patient to elevating and lowering the arm. In ultrasound try to scan for axillary artery which lies at a deeper level. Confirm the artery by color Doppler or pulse wave Doppler.

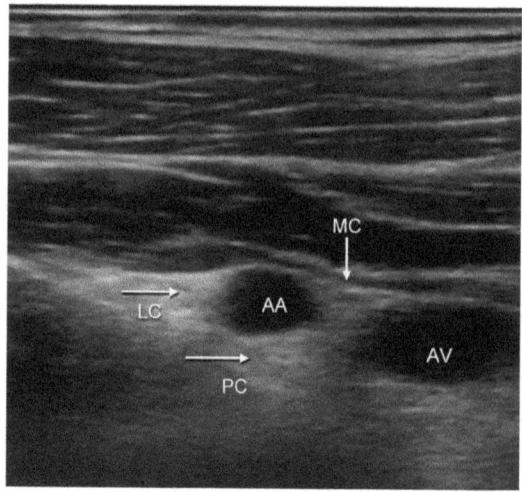

Fig. 12: Ultrasound image of infraclavicular approach of brachial plexus block

Abbreviations: AA, axillary artery; MC, medial cord; LC, lateral cord; PC, posterior cord

Now look for the three cords surrounding the artery. If any doubt please use nerve locator to confirm the cords.

Then insert the needle in plane (Fig. 12) just below the clavicle, first towards the posterior aspect of artery, confirm needle tip by injecting 1 to 2 mL of local anesthetic after negative aspiration. After that inject rest of the local anesthetic volume, around 20 to 30 mL volume is sufficient for successful blockade.

Important note:
- While injecting drug aspirate every 5 mL to decrease a risk of an intravascular injection.
- Do not inject when the resistance to injection is high.
- Do not change the transducer pressure throughout the injection (this can 'open and close' veins in the area and possibly increase the risk of an intravascular injection).

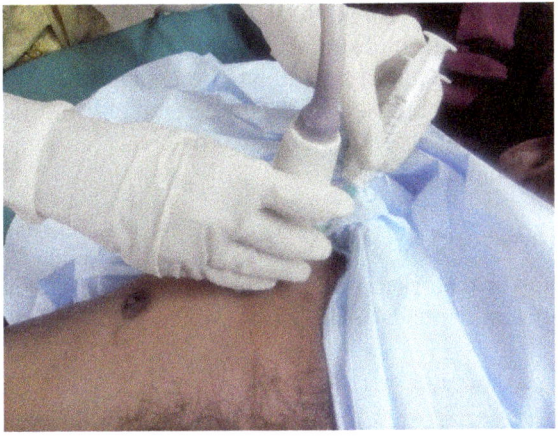

Fig. 13: Probe position for infraclavicular approach of brachial plexus block

ULTRASOUND-GUIDED FOREARM BLOCK

General Considerations

Indications

This block is best suited for hand and/or wrist surgery and sometimes as supplementing failed brachial block.

Advantage of Forearm Block

- Individual nerves can be blocked here so selective area can be blocked
- As no major vessel lies here chances of vascular puncture are decreased
- Less volume of local anesthetic is required
- Complications due to brachial plexus blockade can be avoided
- Total volume of local anesthetic required is 20–25 mL

In forearm block three nerves radial, median and ulnar are blocked at different level. It is useful supplements for an incomplete brachial plexus block and can also be used with light general anesthesia to provide prolonged postoperative analgesia after surgery on the hand and forearm.

Ultrasound Anatomy

In forearm block three nerves radial, ulnar, and median nerve individually are blocked at different locations.

Radial Nerve

The structure of interest are biceps muscle, triceps muscle and humerus. The radial nerve can be visualized in the fascia between the brachioradialis and the brachialis muscles above the lateral aspect of the elbow.

Transducer Position

The patient should be in supine position with flexion of the arm and hand should be at patient's abdomen. Place the transducer transversely on the anterolateral aspect of the distal arm, 3-4 cm above the elbow crease. The nerve appears as a hyperechoic, triangular, or oval structure with the characteristic stippled appearance of a distal peripheral nerve (Fig. 14).

Technique for Radial Nerve Blockade in Forearm

After proper positioning and sterile precaution place the transducer as mentioned above. Radial nerve identification is little bit difficult under ultrasound, but try to find out biceps and brachiradialis muscle. Radial nerve will be seen as hyperechoic rim between these two muscles (Fig. 15).

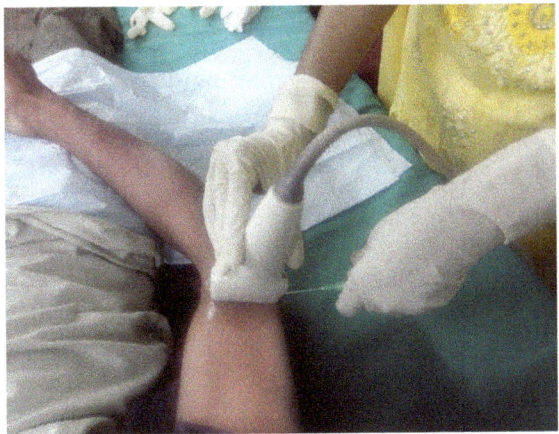

Fig. 14: Probe position for radial nerve block in forearm

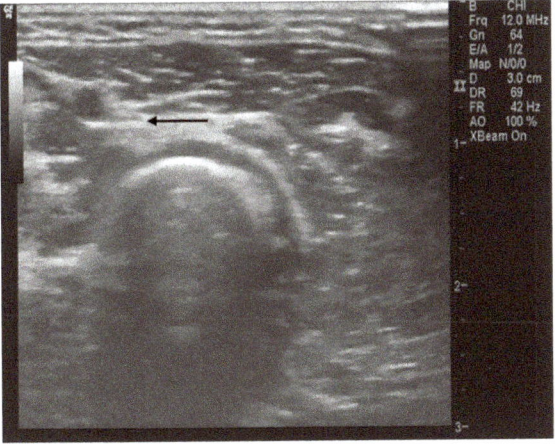

Fig. 15: Arrow shows the radial nerve

Insert the needle in-plane to traverse across the biceps brachii muscle. After negative aspiration confirm the needle tip position by injecting 1 to 2 mL of local anesthetic and then inject 4 to 5 mL of the drug.

Median Nerve

For locating median nerve the most important muscles to visualize are flexor digitorum superficialis, flexor digitorum profundus and palmaris longus muscle. The median nerve will be seen as oval hyperechoic structure between the flexor digitorum superficialis and the flexor palmaris longus muscle.

Technique

- *Patient position:* Supine with arm abducted slightly as per patient's comfort.
- *Transducer position:* Place the transducer transversely in the midforearm on the volar aspect (Fig. 16).

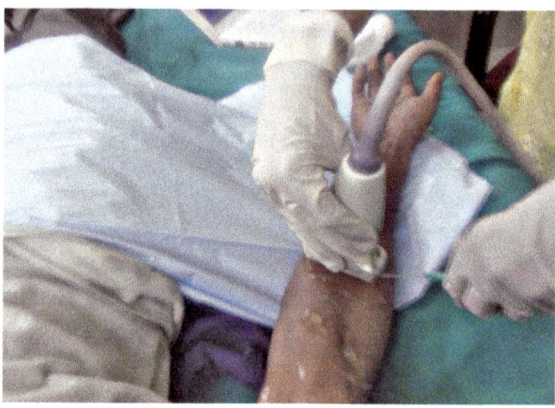

Fig. 16: Probe position for median nerve block in forearm

Upper Extremity Nerve Blocks

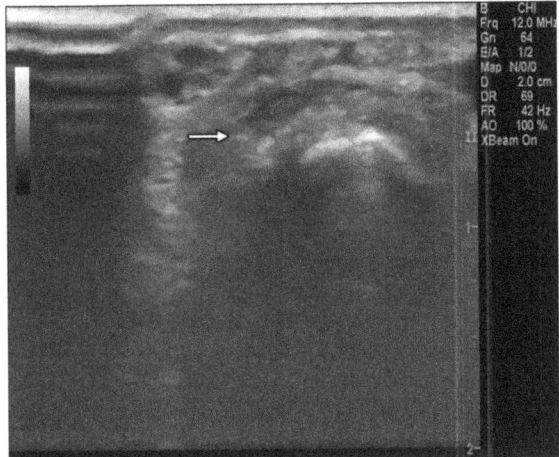

Fig. 17: Arrow shows the median nerve

Technique: After full sterile precaution place the transducer as mentioned above and start scanning. Now initially it will be difficult to locate nerve so move the transducer laterally, find out radial artery using color Doppler and bring the transducer back to midline. The median nerve will be seen approximately 1–2 cm medial and 1 cm deep to the radial artery (Fig. 17).

Then insert the needle in-plane laterally, confirm needle tip with 1 to 2 mL of local anesthetic injection and then after negative aspiration inject rest of the volume that is 4 to 5 mL of local anesthetic.

Ulnar Nerve

The structure of interest are ulnar artery, flexor carpi ulnaris, flexor digitorum profundus muscles and flexor digitorum superficialis muscle. UN appears as a hyperechoic stippled structure, with a triangular to oval shape near to the ulnar artery, sandwiched between the flexor carpi ulnaris and flexor digitorum profundus muscles.

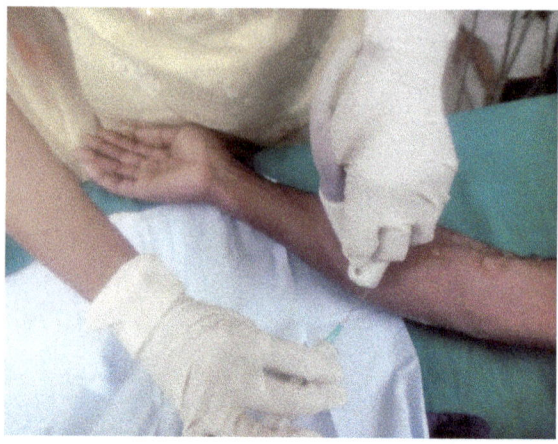

Fig. 18: Probe position for ulnar nerve block in forearm

- *Patient position:* Supine with arm abducted and the palm up.
- *Transducer position (Fig. 18):* Probe position is same as median nerve location but it is medially. As in median nerve here move the transducer medially to find out ulnar artery and confirm with color Doppler. The ulnar nerve lies medial to the artery.

Insert the needle in-plane from medial side confirm needle tip with 1 to 2 mL of local anesthetic injection and then after negative aspiration inject rest of the volume that is 4–5 mL of local anesthetic.

BIBLIOGRAPHY

1. Blaivas M, Lyon M. Ultrasound-guided interscalene block for shoulder dislocation reduction in the ED. Am J Emerg Med. 2006;24(3):293-6.
2. Chan VWS, Perlas A, McCartney CJL, Brull R, Xu D, Abbas S. Ultrasound Guidance Improves Success Rate of Axillary

Brachial Plexus Block. Canadian Journal of Anesthesia. 2007;54:176-82.
3. Chan VWS, Perlas A, Rawson R, Odukoya. Ultrasound-Guided Supraclavicular Brachial Plexus Block. Anesth Analg. 2003;97:1514-7
4. Christophe J-L, Berthier F, Boillot A, Tatu L, Viennet A, Boichut N, et al. Assessment of topographic brachial plexus nerves variations at the axilla using ultrasonography. British Journal of Anaesthesia. 2009;103(4):606-12.
5. Liebmann O, Price D, Mills C, Gardner R, Wang R, Wilson S, et al. Feasibility of Forearm Ultrasound-Guided Nerve Blocks of the Radial, Ulnar and Median Nerves for Hand Procedures in the Emergency Department. Ann Emerg Med. 2006;48(5):558-62.
6. Retzl G, Kapral S, Greher M, Mauritz W. Ultrasonographic Findings of the Axillary Part of the Brachial Plexus. Anesth Analg. 2001;92:1271-5.
7. Sandhu NS, Capan LM. Ultrasound-guided Infraclavicular Brachial Plexus Block. BJA. 2002;89:254-9.
8. Stone MB, Wang R, Price DD. Ultrasound-guided supraclavicular brachial plexus nerve block vs procedural sedation for the treatment of upper extremity emergencies. Am J Emerg Med. 2008;26(6):706-10.
9. Ultrasound guided Axillary nerve block: New York Society of Regional Anaesthesia: 3017 June :2013.
10. Ultrasound guided forearm nerve block: New York Society of Regional Anaesthesia: 3066 August :2013.
11. Ultrasound guided infraclavicular nerve block: New York Society of Regional Anaesthesia: 3016 June :2013.
12. Ultrasound guided interscalene nerve block: New York Society of Regional Anaesthesia: 3014 June :2013.
13. Ultrasound guided supraclavicular nerve block: New York Society of Regional Anaesthesia: 3015 September :2013.
14. Ultrasound guided wrist block: New York Society of Regional Anaesthesia: 3067 September :2013.
15. Wildsmith JAW, Armitage EN, McClure JH. Principles and Practice of Regional Anaesthesia. Third edition. Page no. 193-208.
16. Winnie AP. Interscalene brachial plexus block. Anesth Analg. 1970;49(3):455-66.

Chapter 7

Lower Extremity Nerve Blocks

In this chapter we will discuss about femoral nerve block and popliteal sciatic nerve block under ultrasound guidance.

ULTRASOUND-GUIDED FEMORAL NERVE BLOCK

Anatomy (Fig. 1)

The femoral nerve (L_2-L_4) runs down the posterolateral wall of the pelvis behind the fascia iliaca. The femoral artery and vein lie anterior to the fascia iliaca. As the vessels pass behind the inguinal ligament they become invested in a fascial sheath. The femoral nerve lies behind and lateral to this sheath but is not within it. All three are deep to the fascia lata, but unfortunately the exact position of the nerve in relation to the artery is inconsistent. It may be close to the sheath or several centimeters lateral to it, as well as being more deeply placed. Because of these femoral nerve block is not easy by anatomical landmark technique rather ultrasound is very much helpful to locate the nerve. Ultrasound application helps to monitor the spread of local anesthetic and needle placement and make appropriate adjustments, should the initial spread be deemed inadequate. Also, because of the proximity to the relatively large femoral artery, ultrasound may

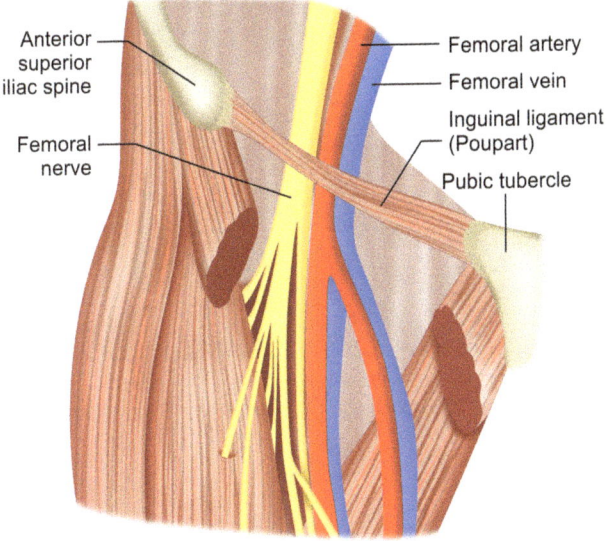

Fig. 1: Anatomy of femoral nerve

reduce the risk of arterial puncture that often occurs with this block with the use of non-ultrasound techniques.

Femoral nerve block results in anesthesia of the anterior and medial thigh down to the knee (the knee included), as well as a variable strip of skin on the medial leg.

Sonoanatomy

The main structure to visualize for femoral nerve block are femoral artery, femoral vein, and fascia iliaca. The femoral artery should be located first using color Doppler and pulse wave Doppler. The femoral vein can be seen medially while femoral nerve will be seen laterally as hyperechoic round or oval rim (Fig. 2).

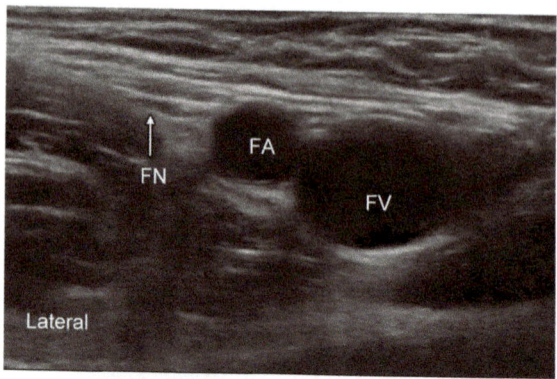

Fig. 2: Sonoanatomy of femoral nerve
Abbreviations: FV, femoral vein; FA, femoral artery; FN, femoral nerve

Indications

- Femoral nerve block is indicated for surgeries on anterior thigh and knee
- For providing postoperative analgesia for surgeries on anterior thigh and knee
- Along with lateral cutaneous nerve of thigh it is indicated for surgeries on thigh and knee
- The total volume required is 20 to 30 mL of local anesthetic.

Patient position: Supine.

Transducer position: Transducer should be placed transversely close to the inguinal crease.

Technique: After proper positioning and sterile precaution place the transducer as mentioned above and start scanning. First of all locate the femoral artery using color Doppler, just above it fascia iliaca can be seen. The femoral nerve lies lateral to artery as hyperechoic rim. If femoral nerve is not visualized tilting and sliding of transducer helps to locate the nerve.

Insert the needle in-plane from lateral to medial side. Once needle tip reaches up to the nerve confirm by injecting 1 to 2 mL of loal anesthetic. After that inject rest of the local anesthetic volume that is 10–20 mL of local anesthetic.

Important Note
When in doubt, the nerve stimulator can also be used along with ultrasound.

Never inject against high resistance to injection because this may signal an intrafascicular needle placement.

ULTRASOUND-GUIDED POPLITEAL SCIATIC NERVE BLOCK

Anatomy of Sciatic Nerve (Fig. 3)

- The sciatic nerve is the larget nerve supplying the leg. It is formed by the fusion of Lumbar fourth, fifth nerves and 3 sacral spinal nerves. It leaves the pelvis through the greater sciatic foramen and runs toward the posterior aspect of the thigh between the greater trochanter and the ischial tuberosity.
- Then it divides into two major branches: (1) Tibial nerve and (2) common peroneal nerve. The tibial nerve supplies the heel and the sole of the foot. The common peroneal, also known as the common fibular nerve, innervates the lateral aspect of the leg and dorsum of the foot.
- At the popliteal crease, the nerves are midway between skin and bone. They are lateral and superficial to the popliteal artery and vein in a separate sheath.
- The tibial nerve is the larger of the two divisions and runs in the middle of popliteal fossa passing inferiorly through the two heads of the gastrocnemius. The common peroneal nerve is more lateral and superficial than the tibial nerve.

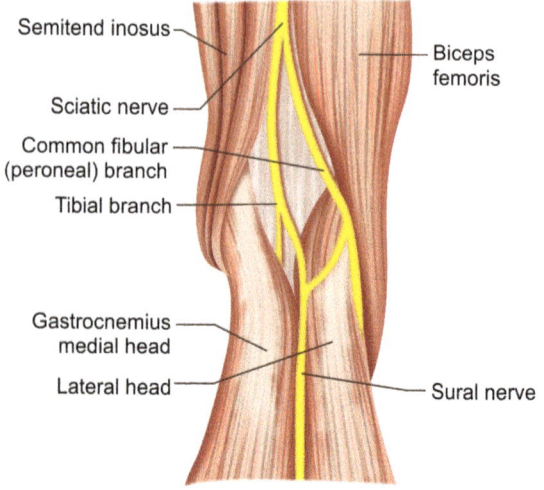

Fig. 3: Popliteal sciatic nerve anatomy

General Considerations

As mentioned above the two branches of sciatic nerve lies deep it is difficult to locate the nerve using anatomical blind technique. So, the ultrasound along with nerve locator is the best way to locate the sciatic popliteal nerve.

There are two approaches for popliteal sciatic block, lateral approach and posterior approach. In both position ultrasound image remains same but the patient position differs.

Position of the Patient

In lateral approach patient position is right or left lateral (more commonly, oblique position) and in posterior approach patient should lie in prone position.

Indications

For operations and postoperative analgesia on lower limb below knee.

Ultrasound Anatomy

The structure of interest are popliteal artery, popliteal vein, biceps femoris muscle and semimembranosus and semitendinosus muscles. The biceps femoris muscle lies lateral to the artery and semi-membranosus and semitendinosus muscles lie medial to the artery. The tibial nerve is seen as a hyperechoic, oval, or round structure with a stippled or honeycomb pattern just superficial and lateral to the artery, while common peroneal nerve is located even more superficial and lateral to the tibial nerve (Fig. 4).

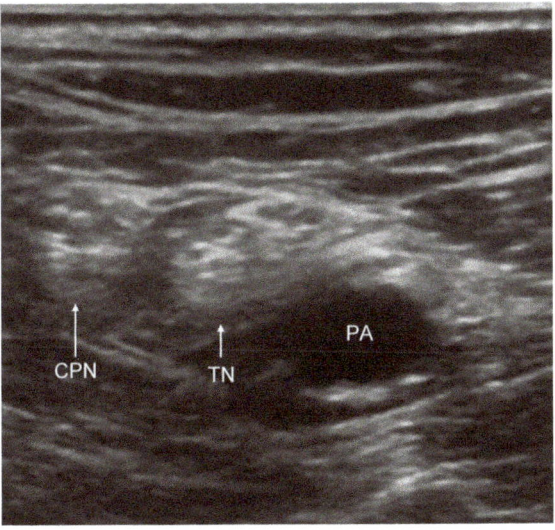

Fig. 4: Sonoanatomy of popliteal sciatic nerve
Abbreviations: PA, popliteal artery; TN, tibial nerve; CPN, common peroneal nerve

Patient's Position

Prone position with the legs slightly abducted. A small footrest is useful to facilitate identification of a motor response if nerve stimulation is used. Also, it relaxes the hamstring tendons, making transducer placement and manipulation easier.

Transducer Position

Transversely at the popliteal crease on the lateral aspect of thigh or over popliteal fossa.

Technique

First of all try to identify popliteal artery, aided with the color Doppler ultrasound when necessary, at a depth of approximately 3-4 cm. The popliteal vein also accompanies the artery.

On either side of the artery are the biceps femoris muscles (lateral) and the semi-membranosus and semitendinosus muscles (medial). Superficially (i.e. toward the skin surface) and lateral to the artery is the tibial nerve, seen as a hyperechoic, oval, or round structure with a stippled or honeycomb pattern on the interior.

If difficulty in identifying the nerve is encountered, the patient can be asked to dorsiflex and plantar flex the ankle, which makes the nerve rotate or move in relation to its surroundings.

Once the tibial nerve is identified, an attempt should be made to visualize the common peroneal nerve, which is located even more superficial and lateral to the tibial nerve. Then move the transducer proximally until the tibial and peroneal nerves are visualized coming together to form the sciatic nerve before its division. This is usually seen at a distance between 5 cm and 10 cm from the popliteal crease, but this may occur very close to the crease or (less commonly) more proximally in the thigh.

As the transducer is moved proximally, the popliteal vessels move anteriorly and therefore become less visible. At all the times keep adjusting depth, gain, and direction of the ultrasound beam to keep the nerve visible. The sciatic nerve typically is visualized at a depth of 2-4 cm.

Once identified, a skin wheal is made immediately lateral or medial to the transducer. Then insert the needle in-plane toward the sciatic nerve.

If nerve stimulation is used (0.5 mA, 0.1 msec), the contact of the needle tip with the sciatic nerve often is associated with a motor response of the calf or foot. Once the needle tip is confirmed to be adjacent to the nerve, inject the local anesthetic after negative aspiration.

Needle repositioning and injection of small aliquots is frequently required to ensure adequate circumferential spread of the local anesthetic.

When injection of the local anesthetic does not appear to result in a spread around the sciatic nerve, additional needle repositions and injections may be necessary. When injecting into the epineurium, correct injection is recognized as local anesthetic spread proximally and distally to the site of the injection around both divisions of the nerve. This typically results in separation of TN and CPN during and after the injection.

Important Note
The nerve stimulator can be useful to confirm the proper placement of needle.

Never inject against high resistance to injection because this may signal an intraneural injection.

BIBLIOGRAPHY

1. Beach ML, Chinn C, et al. A comparison of sensory and motor loss after a femoral nerve block conducted with ultrasound versus ultrasound and nerve stimulation. Reg Anesth Pain Med. 2009;34:508-13.
2. Beaudoin FL, Nagdev A, Merchant RC, Becker BM. Ultrasound-guided femoral nerve blocks in elderly patients with hip fractures. Am J Emerg Med. 2010;28(1):76-81.
3. Gray AT, Huczko EL, Schafhalter-Zoppoth I. Lateral popliteal nerve block with ultrasound guidance. Reg Anesth Pain Med. 2004;29:507-9.
4. McQuay HJ, Carroll D, Moore RA. Postoperative orthopaedic pain: the effect of opiate premedication and local anesthetic blocks. Pain. 1988;33(3):29-5.
5. Schafthalter- Zoppoth I. The "see-saw" sign: improved sonographic identification of the sciatic nerve. Anesthesiology. 2004;101:808-9.
6. Sinha A, Chan VW. Ultrasound imaging for popliteal sciatic nerve block. Reg Anesth Pain Med. 2004;29:130-4.
7. Sites BD, Gallagher JD, Tomek I, Cheung Y, Beach ML. The use of magnetic resonance imaging to evaluate the accuracy of a handheld ultrasound machine in locating the sciatic nerve in the popliteal fossa. Reg Anesth Pain Med. 2004;29:413-6.
8. Ultrasound guided Ankle block: New York Society of Regional Anaesthesia : 3268 September :2013.
9. Ultrasound guided femoral nerve block: New York Society of Regional Anaesthesia: 2013;3267.
10. Ultrasound guided popliteal sciatic nerve block: New York Society of Regional Anaesthesia : 3416 October :2013.
11. Wildsmith JAW, Armitage EN, McClure JH. Principles and practice of regional anaesthesia, 3rd edition. pp. 216-25.

8

Chapter

Transversus Abdominis Plane Block

INTRODUCTION

The transversus abdominis plane block (TAP Block) is a commonly used regional anesthesia technique particularly for postoperive analgesia in different abdominal surgeries. It has been observed that there are minimal complications associated with TAP block. The technique was first described by Rafi in 2001 as a landmark technique. In this technique local anesthtic is being injected between the transversus abdominis and internal oblique muscles.

The TAP block can be given at different level depending on type of surgery. Ultrasound helps to localize exact layers of different abdominal muscles and thus facilitates proper drug distribution between transversus abdominis and internal oblique muscles. Using ultrasound individual nerves like Ilioinguinal and Iliohypogastric can also be blocked.

ANATOMY (FIG. 1)

- Anterolateral abdominal wall is innervated by the nerves arising from the anterior rami of spinal nerves T_7 to L_1 which include the intercostal nerves ($T_7 T_{11}$), the subcostal nerve (T_{12}), and the iliohypogastric and ilioinguinal nerves (L_1). They give rise to the anterior

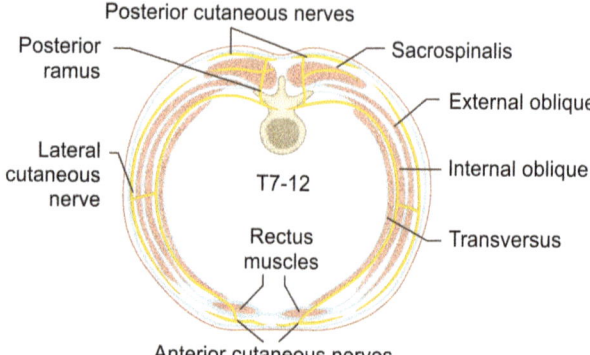

Fig. 1: Transverse section of the abdominal wall showing the path of nerves T7–T12 (Left) and L1 (Right) within the transversus plane

cutaneous and lateral cutaneous branches as they become more superficial.
- The anterior divisions of T_7–T_{11} run in the neurovascular plane in abdominal wall between the internal oblique and transversus abdominis muscles until they reach to the rectus abdominis where they perforate and supply, ending as anterior cutaneous branches supplying the skin of the front of the abdomen. In their course they pierce the external oblique muscle midway giving off the lateral cutaneous branch which divides into anterior and posterior branches that supply the external oblique muscle and latissimus dorsi respectively. The anterior branch of T_{12} communicates with the iliohypogastric nerve and gives a branch to the pyramidalis. Its lateral cutaneous branch perforates the internal and external oblique muscles and descends over the iliac crest and supplies sensation to the front part of the gluteal region.

Transversus Abdominis Plane Block

- T-6 to T-12 provide sensory innervation to the skin, costal part of diaphragm, related partial pleura and peritoneum. T-7 gives sensory innervation at epigastrium, at umbilicus and L-1 at the groin.
- Division of the iliohypogastric nerve (L1) occurs between the internal oblique and transversus abdominis near the iliac crest giving rise to lateral and anterior cutaneous branches, the former supplying part of the skin of the gluteal region while the latter supplies the hypogastric region.
- The ilioinguinal nerve (L1) communicates with the iliohypogastric nerve between the internal oblique and transversus abdominis near the anterior part of the iliac crest. It supplies the upper and medial part of the thigh and part of the skin covering the genitalia.

Thus, in TAP block we deposit local anesthetic in plane between the internal oblique and transversus abdominis muscle. It mainly blocks the abdominal skin, muscles and parietal peritoneum, **so dull visceral pain remains present even after TAP block.**

INDICATIONS

- To provide Postoperative pain relief in lower abdominal surgeries like appendectomy, hernia repair, cesarean section, abdominal hysterectomy, prostatectomy.
- Bilateral blocks can be given for midline incisions or laparoscopic surgery. Care should be taken not to exceed recommended safe doses of local anesthetic agent with bilateral injections.
- Subcostal TAP block is given just beneath the costal margin to provide postoperative analgesia for supraumbilical surgeries.

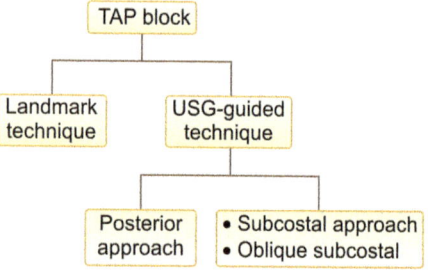

THE LANDMARK TECHNIQUE FOR TAP BLOCK

For blind technique of TAP block needle should be inserted from the lumbar triangle of petit, which lies between lower costal margin and iliac crest. Anatomically external oblique muscle lies anterior to it and latissimus dorsi lies posterior to it. In blind technique after inserting needle two resistance of external and internal oblique muscles are felt.

ULTRASOUND GUIDED TAP BLOCK

Advantages

Under ultrasound guidance we can differentiate all the abdominal layers, so that accurate placement of the drug can be confirmed.

ULTRASOUND ANATOMY

All the layers of abdominal wall can be recognized under ultrasound guidance. Thus as we go from superficial to deep skin, subcutaneous tissue, fat, external oblique, internal oblique, transversus abdominis muscle can be seen. The peritoneum and bowel loops can be recognized deep to the muscles.

Sonoanatomy of TAP Block (Fig. 2)

After proper positioning and sterile precaution place the transducer as described above, and start scanning. In ultrasound. The three muscle layers can be seen as a hyperechoic fascia, the outermost external oblique (EOM), the internal oblique (IOM), and the transverses abdominis muscles (TAM). Immediately below this last muscle is the transversalis fascia, followed by the peritoneum and the intestines below, which can be recognized as moving structures because of peristalsis. The nerves of the abdominal wall cannot be visualized. Imaging of the abdominal wall between the costal margin and the iliac crest reveals three muscle layers.

Patient Position

Supine or lateral position with the arm on the side to be blocked elevated and turned to the opposite side.

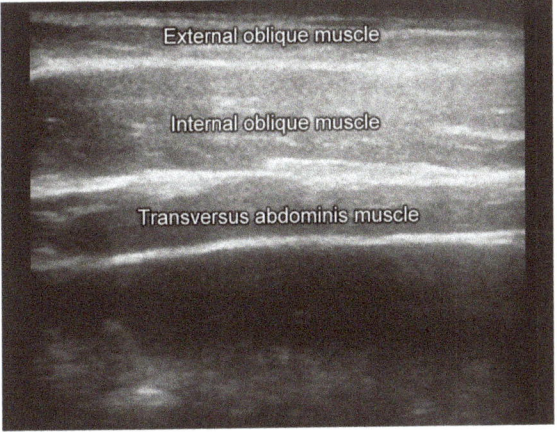

Fig. 2: Sonoanatomy of transverese abdominis plane

Type of Transduser

A broad linear array ultrasound probe (8–14 Hz frequency) is used with an imaging depth of 4–6 cm.

Scanning

The ultrasound probe is placed transverse to the abdomen (horizontal plane) in the mid-axillary line between the costal margin and the iliac crest. 3 muscle layer will be clearly seen in the image (posterior approach).

Transducer Position

The position of transducer depends upon the type of surgery (Fig. 3).

1. *Transducer position for lower abdominal surgeries:* For providing postoperative analgesia for surgeries like laparotomy, appendicectomy, abdominoplasty, and cesarean delivery the transducer shoud be placed between the costal margin and the iliac crest at the anterior axillary line. Transducer should be kept transversely on the abdomen. The drug should be deposited between the transversus abdominis and internal oblique muscle planes.

   The volume of local anesthetic required is 20–30 mL. Needle required is long needle of at least 5–8 cm length.

2. *Transducer position for inguinal region surgeries:* For postoperative analgesia for inguinal hernia repair and other inguinal surgery the position of transducer should be kept on a line joining the anterior superior iliac spine (ASIS) with the umbilicus or as posterior approach. The goal is to spread local anesthetic between the transversus abdominis and internal oblique muscle planes, in the vicinity of the two nerves. The volume required is 10–20 mL each side.

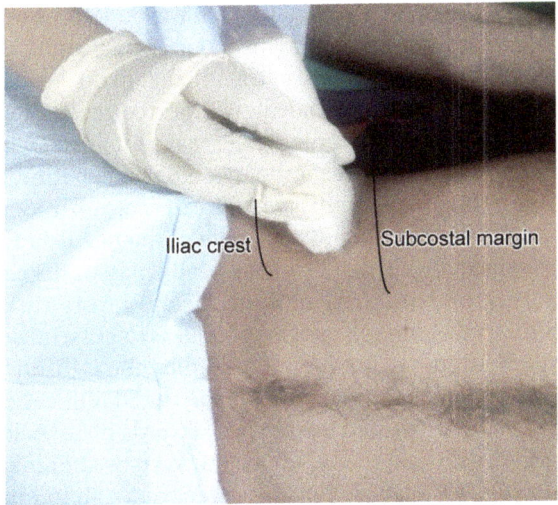

Fig. 3: Transducer position for TAP block in inguinal region

3. *Transducer position for upper abdominal surgeries:* For postoperative analgesia for umbilical hernia repair and other umbilical surgery the transducer should be placed transversely on abdomen, immediately lateral to umbilicus. The goal is to deposit local anesthetic between rectus muscle and posterior rectus sheath local anesthetic required is 10 ml per side.

Type of Needle

18 or 20 G Toughy needle or 22 g stimuplex with the length of 5-8 cm can be used.

TECHNIQUE OF TAP BLOCK

After proper positioning and sterile precaution place the transducer as described above, and start scanning. The needle is to be inserted in a sagittal plane with bevel facing up just medial to the ultrasound probe (in plane technique) (Fig. 4). For better visualization, the needle should be directed perpendicular to the beam of ultrasound waves. When needle will be in correct position in transversus abdominis plane, real time ultrasound imaging allows observation of needle passage through the skin, subcutaneous tissue then external and internal oblique muscles. On advancement of the needle a two pop sensation can be elicited as needle passes through external and internal oblique fascial layers (as in landmark technique). Internal oblique is thickest muscle layer. If layers are not identified sliding the transducer slightly cephalad or caudad will aid the identification. The needle tip should be directed towards plane below the internal oblique and above transverses abdominis muscle (TAP plane). Once the transverse abdominal plane is identified, infiltrate 1–2 mL of local anesthetic to form skin wheel and insert the needle in plane (Fig. 5). After gentle aspiration, inject 1–2 mL of local anesthetic to verify the location of the needle tip. When injection

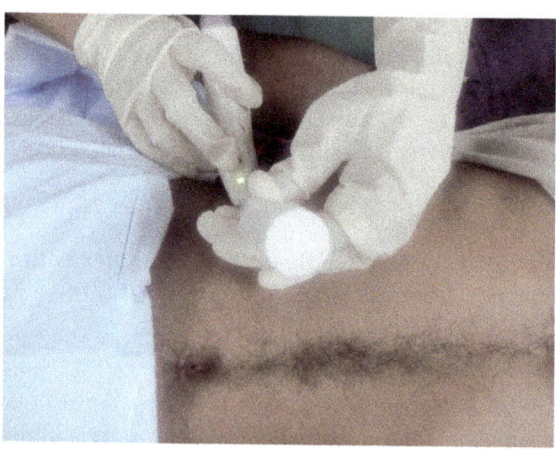

Fig. 4: Technique of needle insertion

Transversus Abdominis Plane Block

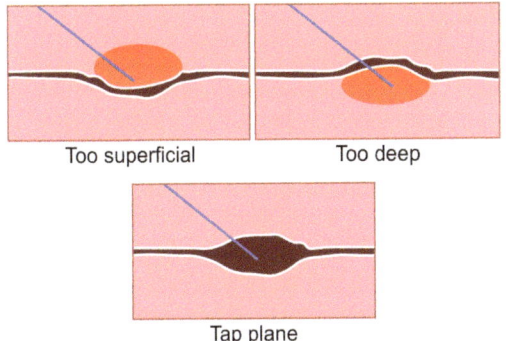

Fig. 5: Needle tip position

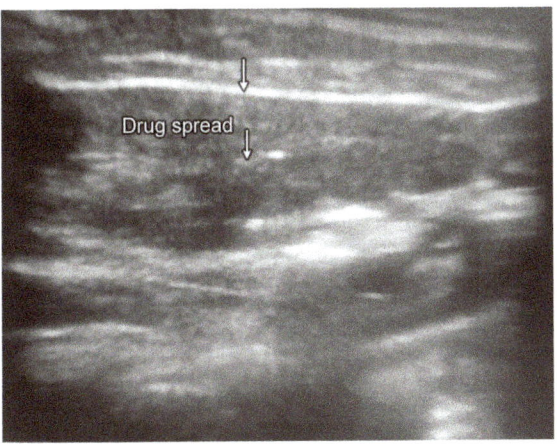

Fig. 6: Spread of drug in transverese abdominis plane

of the local anesthetic appears to be intramuscular, the needle is advanced or withdrawn carefully 1–2 mm and another bolus is administered. This gesture is repeated until the correct plane is achieved. In an adult patient, 20 mL of local anesthetic per side is usually sufficient for successful blockade. Figure 6 shows the spread of drug.

Technique

After proper positioning and sterile precaution place the tranducer as described above, and start scanning. The three muscle layers separated by a hyperechoic fascia, the outermost external oblique (EOM), the internal oblique (IOM), and the transversus abdominis muscles (TAM) will be seen. Immediately below this last muscle is the transversalis fascia, followed by the peritoneum and the intestines below, which can be recognized as moving structures because of peristalsis. The nerves of the abdominal wall cannot be visualized. Imaging of the abdominal wall between the costal margin and the iliac crest reveals three muscle layers.

Needle Insertion

The needle is to be inserted in a sagittal plane with bevel facing up just medial to the ultrasound probe (in plane technique). For better visualization, the needle should be directed perpendicular to the beam of ultrasound waves. When needle will be in correct position in transversus abdominis plane, real time ultrasound imaging allows observation of needle passage through the skin, subcutaneous tissue then external and internal oblique muscles. The needle tip should be directed towards plane below the internal oblique and above transversus abdominis muscle (TAP plane). Drug should be injected here.

Identifying the TAP Plane

Once the transverse abdominal plane is identified, infiltrate 1-2 mL of local anesthetic to form skin wheel and insert the needle in plane. On advancement of the needle a two pop sensation can be elicited as needle passes through external and internal oblique fascial layers (as in landmark technique).Internal oblique is thickest muscle layer. If layers are not identified sliding the transducer slightly cephalad or caudad will aid the identification.. After gentle aspiration, inject 1 to 2 mL of local anesthetic to verify the location of the needle tip. When injection of the local anesthetic appears to be intramuscular, the needle is advanced or withdrawn carefully 1-2 mm and another bolus is administered. This gesture is repeated until the correct plane is achieved. In an adult patient, 20 mL of local anesthetic per side is usually sufficient for successful blockade.

COMPLICATIONS

Chances of complications are very less with TAP block still there are rare chances of intrahepatic injection with subcostal approach likely complications are as follows:
- Intrahepatic injection with subcostal approach
- Intraperitoneal injection
- Bowel hematoma
- Transient femoral nerve palsy.

Local anesthetic toxicity could also occur due to the large volumes required to perform this block especially if it was done bilaterally.

As with any regional technique, careful aspiration will help avoid intravascular injections though Tap plane is hypovascular.

BIBLIOGRAPHY

1. Moore K, Dalley A. Clinically Oriented Anaomy, 5th edition. Philadelphia: Lippincott Williams and Wilkins, 2006:206.
2. Snell R. Clinical anatomy 8th edition Baltimore. Lippincott Williams and Wilkins, 2008.
3. Tammam TF. Transversus abdominis plane block: The analgesic efficacy of a new block catheter insertion

method. Egyptian Journal of Anaesthesia. 2014;30(1): 39–45.
4. Tran TMN, Ivanusic JJ, Hebbard P, Barrington MJ. Determination of spread of injectate after ultrasound guided transerversus abdominis plane block: a cadaveric study. Br J Anaesth. 2009;102:123-7.
5. Ultrasound guided TAP block: New York Society of regional Anaesthesia, September 2013.

Index

Page numbers followed by *f* refer to figure

A
Abdominal wall, transverse section of 120*f*
Acoustic shadow bone 13*f*
Air embolism, prevention of 62
Alternative central venous cannulation sites 49
Amides 77
Anechoic vein 27*f*
Ankle block 85
Antecubital region, major vessels of 69*f*
Antimicrobial-impregnated catheters 59
Antiseptic solution 22
Arterial
 access procedures 72
 flow 29
 puncture 57, 61
  recognition of 62
 trauma 24
  management of 62
 wall 30*f*
Arteries 9*f*, 30
 axillary 98, 100, 102
Arteriovenous fistula 57
Atropine 82
Axillary block 97, 99*f*

B
Bier's block 78
Bladder perforation 57
Bleeding disorders 19
Blood clot 57
Bloodstream infection, catheter-related 60
B-mode 8
Bone 15
Bowel hematoma 129
Brachial plexus 91, 92, 92*f*, 94, 96, 98*f*
 anatomy of 87, 88*f*
 block 87, 96*f*, 102*f*, 103*f*
  axillary approach of 100*f*
 organization of 89*f*
 sonoanatomy of 94*f*
 ultrasound anatomy of 91*f*
Brachial vein 69*f*
 cannulation 69*f*
Brachiocephalic vein 34, 45*f*
Brightness mode 8
Bupivacaine 77
Burns 19

C

Cannulate peripheral veins 66
Cardiac arrest 19
Carotid artery 91, 92
Cartilage 15
Catheter
  fixation technique 23
  insertion site, selection of 22, 23
  knotting 57
  maintenance 23, 60
  malposition 61
  placement 24
  types of 59
Cellulitis 19, 32, 57
Central processing unit 3, 5
Central venous
  access 16
    complications of 57
  catheterization 24, 58*f*, 62
    complications of 48
  pressure 16
Cephalic vein 69*f*
  cannulation 70*f*
Chest radiography 24
Chloroprocaine 77
Computer central processing unit 5

D

Deep vein thrombosis 33, 61
Dermatitis, severe 19
Disc storage device 4
Doppler ultrasound 8
Dysrhythmias 57

E

Edema, severe 19
Electrocardiogram 82
Ephedrine 82
Epidural anesthesia 77
External jugular vein 50

F

Fascia 15
Faster performance time 84
Fat 15
Femoral
  artery 112
  nerve 110, 112
    anatomy of 111*f*
    block 85
    sonoanatomy of 112*f*
  vein 34, 45, 61, 112
    anatomy 46*f*
    cannulation, technique for 48
    sonoanatomy of 47*f*
    venipuncture 48
    venous route 48
Forearm block 84, 103

H

Hematoma 57, 61, 81
Hemomediastinum 57
Hemothorax 19, 57
Hydrothorax 57
Hypertension 76

I

Iliohypogastric nerve, division of 121
Infection 61, 81
Inferior petrosal sinus 34
Infiltration anesthesia 77
Inguinal region 125*f*
  surgeries, transducer position for 124
Innominate vein 34, 43
Internal carotid artery 34

Internal jugular vein 33, 34, 61
  cannulation 35
    technique for 36
  left 49
Internal jugular vessels,
    anatomy of 35*f*
Intrahepatic injection 129
Intraperitoneal injection 129
Intravenous antibiotic
    prophylaxis, use of 22

J

Jugular foramen 34

L

Landmark technique 82
Levobupivacaine 77
Lidocaine 77
Linear transducer probe 5*f*
Local anesthetic agents 76, 77
Low frequency transducers 10
Lower abdominal surgeries,
    transducer position for
    124
Lower extremity nerve blocks
    110
Lungs 15
Lymph nodes 15

M

Machine, parts of 3*f*
Mechanical trauma,
    prevention of 23
Median nerve 98, 100, 106,
    106*f*, 107*f*
Mental status 82
Mepivacaine 77
Midazolam 83
Middle scalene muscle 91, 92
Mid-range transducers 10
M-mode 7, 8

Morbid obesity 19
Motion mode 8
Multiple previous blind
    catheterizations 19
Muscle 15
  relaxant 83
Musculocutaneous nerve 98,
    100

N

Needle
  insertion 24, 128
    technique of 126*f*
  tip position 127*f*
  types of 125
Nerve 15
  blocks, quality of 84
  damage 81
  injury 57
  localization, optimization of
    84, 86
  path of 120*f*
Non-invasive blood pressure
    82

O

One-person technique 32

P

Pentoxifylline 33
Peripheral nerve
  block 78
  locator technique 82
Peripheral venous access 66
  technique for 70
Peripheral vessels 30
Peroneal nerve 115
Phenylephrine 82
Plexus anesthesia 78
Pneumothorax 61
  contralateral 19

Popliteal artery 115
Popliteal sciatic nerve
  anatomy 114f
  sonoanatomy of 115f
Posterior cord 102
Pressure 11
Procaine 77
Prophylactic antibiotics 59
Propofol 83
Pulse
  oximetry 82
  wave Doppler 9f, 31f
Pythagoras's theorem 38f

R

Radial nerve 98, 100, 104, 105f
  block 105f
    technique for 104
Refraction artifact 13
Regional anesthesia 78
  advantages of 78
  complications of 79
  disadvantages of 79
Respiratory rate 82
Ropivacaine 77

S

Scalene muscle, anterior 91
Sciatic
  nerve, anatomy of 113
  popliteal nerve block 85
Sepsis 57
Shock 19
Single-lumen and multilumen catheters 60
Skull 34
Spinal anesthesia 77
Staphylococcus epidermidis 60
Static method 31

Sternocleidomastoid muscle 35, 91, 92
Subclavian
  artery 94, 96
  vein 34, 43, 46f, 61
    technique for 44
  vessels, anatomy of 35f
Superior iliac spine, anterior 124
Supraclavicular
  approach 44, 84, 88
  block 95f
  level 94f
Surface anesthesia 77

T

TAP block
  sonoanatomy of 123
  technique of 125
Tetracaine 77
Thiopentone sodium 83
Thrombolytic therapy 19
Thrombotic complications 63
Tibial nerve 115
Time gain compensation 6
Transducer
  pulse controls 3, 5
  types of 4f, 124
Transient femoral nerve palsy 129
Transversus abdominis
  muscle 123, 126, 128
  plane 127f
    block 119
    sonoanatomy of 123f
Trendelenburg position 36
Two-dimensional imaging 7
Two-person technique 32

U

Ulnar nerve 98, 100, 107, 108f

Ultrasound 1
  advantages of 2, 17, 83
  anatomy 90, 94, 97, 101, 104, 115, 122
  basics of 1
  disadvantages of 2, 84
  guidance 58, 71
  knobology 5
  machine 3*f*
    knobology of 6*f*
    parts of 3
  terminology 14
  types of 7
Ultrasound guided
  arterial access, technique for 73
  axillary block 96
  central venous access 16
  femoral nerve block 110
  forearm block 103
  infraclavicular brachial plexus block 100
  interscalene brachial plexus block 89
  lower extremity nerve blocks 85
  peripheral venous access 66, 70
    technique for 68
  peripherally inserted central catheter placement, technique for 72
  popliteal sciatic nerve block 113
  regional block 75, 83
  supraclavicular block 93
  TAP block 122
  technique 82
  upper extremity nerve blocks 84
  vascular access 25
    line placement 34
Upper abdominal surgeries, transducer position for 125
Upper extremity nerve blocks 86

V

Vasculitis 19
Veins 29
Vessel 15

W

Wrist block 84

EU GSPR Authorised Reprsentative
Logos Europe, 9 rue Nicolas Poussin
1700, La Rochelle, France
Phone: +33 (0) 6 67 93 73 78
E-mail: contact@logoseurope.eu

www.ingramcontent.com/pod-product-compliance
Ingram Content Group UK Ltd.
Pitfield, Milton Keynes, MK11 3LW, UK
UKHW021827140426
5217IPUK00016B/1232